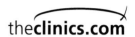

UROLOGIC CLINICS

OF NORTH AMERICA

New Developments in Infection
and Inflammation in Urology

GUEST EDITOR
J. Curtis Nickel, MD

CONSULTING EDITOR
Martin I. Resnick, MD

February 2008 • Volume 35 • Number 1

SAUNDERS

An Imprint of Elsevier, Inc.
PHILADELPHIA   LONDON   TORONTO   MONTREAL   SYDNEY   TOKYO

W.B. SAUNDERS COMPANY
A Division of Elsevier Inc.

1600 John F. Kennedy Boulevard • Suite 1800 • Philadelphia, Pennsylvania 19103-2899

http://www.theclinics.com

UROLOGIC CLINICS OF NORTH AMERICA	**Volume 35, Number 1**
February 2008	**ISSN 0094-0143**
Editor: Kerry Holland	**ISBN-13: 978-1-4160-5844-1**
	ISBN-10: 1-4160-5844-3

Reprints. For copies of 100 or more, of articles in this publication, please contact the Commercial Reprints Department, Elsevier Inc., 360 Park Avenue South, New York, New York 10010-1710. Tel.: (212) 633-3813, Fax: (212) 462-1935, e-mail: reprints@elsevier.com.

The ideas and opinions expressed in *Urologic Clinics of North America* do not necessarily reflect those of the Publisher. The Publisher does not assume any responsibility for any injury and/or damage to persons or property arising out of or related to any use of the material contained in this periodical. The reader is advised to check the appropriate medical literature and the product information currently provided by the manufacturer of each drug to be administered to verify the dosage, the method and duration of administration, or contraindications. It is the responsibility of the treating physician or other health care professional, relying on independent experience and knowledge of the patient, to determine drug dosages and the best treatment for the patient. Mention of any product in this issue should not be construed as endorsement by the contributors, editors, or the Publisher of the product or manufacturers' claims.

Urologic Clinics of North America (ISSN 0094-0143) is published quarterly by Elsevier Inc., 360 Park Avenue South, New York, NY 10010-1710. Months of issue are February, May, August, and November. Business and Editorial Offices: 1600 John F. Kennedy Blvd., Suite 1800, Philadelphia, PA 19103-2899. Customer Service Office: 6277 Sea Harbor Drive, Orlando, FL 32887-4800. Periodicals postage paid at New York, NY and additional mailing offices. Subscription prices are $249.00 per year (US individuals), $394.00 per year (US institutions), $285.00 per year (Canadian individuals), $472.00 per year (Canadian institutions), $333.00 per year (foreign individuals), and $472.00 per year (foreign institutions). Foreign air speed delivery is included in all *Clinics* subscription prices. All prices are subject to change without notice. **POSTMASTER:** Send address changes to *Urologic Clinics of North America*, Elsevier Periodicals Customer Service, 6277 Sea Harbor Drive, Orlando, FL 32887-4800. **Customer Service: 1-800-654-2452 (US). From outside the US, call 1-407-345-4000.**

Urologic Clinics of North America is covered in *Index Medicus, Excerpta Medica, Current Contents/ Clinical Medicine, Science Citation Index,* and *ISI/BIOMED.*

Printed in the United States of America.

CONSULTING EDITOR

MARTIN I. RESNICK, MD,[†] Lester Persky Professor and Chairman, Department of Urology, Case Medical Center, Cleveland, Ohio

GUEST EDITOR

J. CURTIS NICKEL, MD, Professor of Urology, Department of Urology, Queen's University, Kingston, Ontario, Canada

CONTRIBUTORS

ROSS BAUER, MD, Resident, Division of Urology, Department of Urology, Albany Medical College, Albany, New York

BRIAN M. BENWAY, MD, Resident, Division of Urology, Clinical Science Center, University of Wisconsin Hospital-Medical School, Madison, Wisconsin

RAYMOND COSTABILE, MD, Associate Professor of Urology, University of Virginia School of Medicine; and Jay Y. Gillenwater Professor of Surgery and Vice Chairman of Urologic Surgery, University of Virginia, Department of Urology, University of Virginia School of Medicine, Charlottesville, Virginia

TARA LEE FRENKL, MD, MPH, Adjunct Assistant Professor, Division of Urology, University of Pennsylvania, Philadelphia, Pennsylvania

PATTI A. GROOME, PhD, Department of Community Health and Epidemiology, Queen's University, Kingston, Canada; Division of Cancer Care and Epidemiology, Queen's Cancer Research Institute, Queen's University, Kingston, Ontario, Canada

PHILIP M. HANNO, MD, MPH, Professor of Surgery in Urology, Hospital of the University of Pennsylvania, Philadelphia, Pennsylvania

BARRY A. KOGAN, MD, Falk Chair in Urology, Chief, Division of Urology, Department of Urology, Albany Medical College, Albany, New York

STEVE LEBOVITCH, MD, Resident, Department of Urology, Temple University Hospital, Philadelphia, Pennsylvania

TIMOTHY D. MOON, MBChB, FRCSC, Professor of Surgery, Division of Urology, Department of Surgery, University of Wisconsin Hospital-Medical School; and Veterans Affairs Medical Center, Clinical Science Center, Madison, Wisconsin

JACK H. MYDLO, MD, Chairperson, Department of Urology, Temple University Hospital, Philadelphia, Pennsylvania

K.G. NABER, MD, PhD, Professor of Urology, Technical University of Munich, Straubing, Germany

DURWOOD E. NEAL, Jr, MD, Professor and Chief, Division of Urology, Department of Surgery, University of Missouri, Columbia, Missouri

[†] Deceased

J. CURTIS NICKEL, MD, Professor of Urology, Department of Urology, Queen's University, Kingston, Ontario, Canada

LINDSAY E. NICOLLE, MD, FRCPC, Professor, Departments of Internal Medicine and Medical Microbiology, Health Sciences Centre, University of Manitoba, Winnipeg, Canada

MICHEL A. PONTARI, MD, Professor of Urology, Department of Urology, Temple University School of Medicine, Philadelphia, Pennsylvania

JEANNETTE POTTS, MD, Professional Medical Staff, Glickman Urological and Kidney Institute, Cleveland Clinic Foundation, Cleveland, Ohio

D. ROBERT SIEMENS, MD, FRCSC, Department of Anatomy and Cell Biology, Queen's University, Kingston, Canada; Department of Urology, Kingston General Hospital, Queen's University, Kingston, Ontario, Canada

WILLIAM D. STEERS, MD, Professor of Urologic Surgery, University of Virginia School of Medicine; and Hovey Dabney Chair of Urologic Surgery, University of Virginia, Department of Urology, University of Virginia School of Medicine, Charlottesville, Virginia

DAVID STOCK, MSc, Department of Community Health and Epidemiology, Queen's University, Kingston, Canada; Division of Cancer Care and Epidemiology, Queen's Cancer Research Institute, Queen's University, Kingston, Ontario, Canada

CHAD R. TRACY, MD, Chief Urology Resident, Department of Urology, University of Virginia School of Medicine, Charlottesville, Virginia

F.M.E. WAGENLEHNER, MD, PhD, Consultant of Urology, Clinic of Urology and Pediatric Urology, Justus-Liebig-University, Giessen, Germany

W. WEIDNER, MD, PhD, Professor of Urology, Clinic of Urology and Pediatric Urology, Justus-Liebig-University, Giessen, Germany

CONTRIBUTORS

CONTENTS

GOAL STATEMENT

The goal of *Urologic Clinics of North America* is to keep practicing urologists and urology residents up to date with current clinical practice in urology by providing timely articles reviewing the state of the art in patient care.

ACCREDITATION

The *Urologic Clinics of North America* is planned and implemented in accordance with the Essential Areas and Policies of the Accreditation Council for Continuing Medical Education (ACCME) through the joint sponsorship of the University of Virginia School of Medicine and Elsevier. The University of Virginia School of Medicine is accredited by the ACCME to provide continuing medical education for physicians.

The University of Virginia School of Medicine designates this educational activity for a maximum of *15 AMA PRA Category 1 Credits™*. Physicians should only claim credit commensurate with the extent of their participation in the activity.

The American Medical Association has determined that physicians not licensed in the US who participate in this CME activity are eligible for *15 AMA PRA Category 1 Credits™*.

Credit can be earned by reading the text material, taking the CME examination online at http://www.theclinics.com/home/cme, and completing the evaluation. After taking the test, you will be required to review any and all incorrect answers. Following completion of the test and evaluation, your credit will be awarded and you may print your certificate.

FACULTY DISCLOSURE/CONFLICT OF INTEREST

The University of Virginia School of Medicine, as an ACCME accredited provider, endorses and strives to comply with the Accreditation Council for Continuing Medical Education (ACCME) Standards of Commercial Support, Commonwealth of Virginia statutes, University of Virginia policies and procedures, and associated federal and private regulations and guidelines on the need for disclosure and monitoring of proprietary and financial interests that may affect the scientific integrity and balance of content delivered in continuing medical education activities under our auspices.

The University of Virginia School of Medicine requires that all CME activities accredited through this institution be developed independently and be scientifically rigorous, balanced and objective in the presentation/discussion of its content, theories and practices.

All authors/editors participating in an accredited CME activity are expected to disclose to the readers relevant financial relationships with commercial entities occurring within the past 12 months (such as grants or research support, employee, consultant, stock holder, member of speakers bureau, etc.). The University of Virginia School of Medicine will employ appropriate mechanisms to resolve potential conflicts of interest to maintain the standards of fair and balanced education to the reader. Questions about specific strategies can be directed to the Office of Continuing Medical Education, University of Virginia School of Medicine, Charlottesville, Virginia.

The authors/editors listed below have identified no professional or financial affiliations for themselves or their spouse/partner:
Ross Bauer, MD; Brian M. Benway, MD; Patti A. Groome, PhD; Philip M. Hanno, MD, MPH; Kerry K. Holland (Acquisitions Editor); Barry A. Kogan, MD; Steve Lebovitch, MD; Jack Mydlo, MD; Durwood E. Neal, Jr., MD; Lindsay E. Nicolle, MD, FRCPC; D. Robert Siemens, MD, FRCSC; David Stock, MSc; Chad R. Tracy, MD; Florian Martin Erich Wagenlehner, MD, PhD; and, Wolfgang Weidner, MD, PhD.

The authors/editors listed below identified the following professional or financial affiliations for themselves or their spouse/partner:
Raymond Costabile, MD is an independent contractor for Boehringer Ingelheim, and is an independent contractor, consultant, and serves on the Speaker's Bureau for Lilly.
Tara Lee Frenkl, MD, MPH is employed by, owns stock in, and is a patent holder for Merck & Co., Inc, and her spouse is employed by and owns stock in GlaxoSmithKline, Inc.
Timothy D. Moon, MBChB, FRCSC serves on the Advisory Committee for Boehringer Ingelheim.
Kurt G. Naber, MD, PhD serves on the Advisory Board for Basiliea and is a consultant for Bayer, MerLion, Peninsula/Johnson & Johnson, Sanofi Aventis, and Zambon.
J. Curtis Nickel, MD (Guest Editor) is a consultant for Merck Frosst Canada, GSK, Sanofi Aventis, Ortho McNeil, Plethora Solutions, and American Medical Systems, and serves on the Advisory Board for Merck Frosst Canada, GSK, Sanofi Aventis, Ortho McNeil, Bonston Scientific, Allergan, Farr Laboratories, Triton Pharma, and American Medical Systems.
Michel A. Pontari, MD is an independent contractor and serves on the Advisory Board for Pfizer.
Jeanette Potts, MD serves on the Speaker's Bureau and Advisory Committee for Pfizer.
William D. Steers, MD is an independent contractor for Astellas, Allergan, and Pfizer and is a consultant for Astellas, Allergan, Dynogen, and Pfizer.

Disclosure of Discussion of non-FDA approved uses for pharmaceutical products and/or medical devices:
The University of Virginia School of Medicine, as an ACCME provider, requires that all faculty presenters identify and disclose any "off label" uses for pharmaceutical and medical device products. The University of Virginia School of Medicine recommends that each physician fully review all the available data on new products or procedures prior to instituting them with patients.

TO ENROLL

To enroll in the Urologic Clinics of North America Continuing Medical Education program, call customer service at 1-800-654-2452 or visit us online at www.theclinics.com/home/cme. The CME program is available to subscribers for an additional fee of $195.00.

FORTHCOMING ISSUES

ELSEVIER
SAUNDERS

Urol Clin N Am 35 (2008) xi

UROLOGIC
CLINICS
of North America

Preface

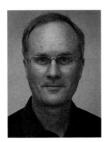

J. Curtis Nickel, MD
Guest Editor

Infection continues to be the most unglamorous and, for most practicing urologists, the most uninteresting topic in our profession. Yet we deal with infection—prevention, diagnosis and management—every day in our clinical practice. Our knowledge on the subject, compared with such exciting topics as prostate cancer, is rudimentary, and for many urologists their grasp of the subject has not changed since their days of residency. Even at that time in our careers, infection questions on the American Board of Urology examinations have always been the most poorly answered of all the urology topics.

Genitourinary syndromes believed to be related to inflammation (not necessarily infectious) are even more of an enigma to urologists. Yet again, multiple surveys have confirmed that conditions such as prostatitis, interstitial cystitis, and related syndromes continue to occupy a significant percentage of our outpatient clinical practice time. Inflammation may also hold the key to the pathogenesis and progression of other, more interesting clinical conditions, such as benign prostatic hyperplasia and even prostate cancer.

Urologists have always prided themselves on keeping up with the latest developments in our field and practicing a best-evidence approach to the management of urologic disease. This issue of *Urologic Clinics of North America* provides an up-to-date contemporary foundation for that strategy on the topic of infection and inflammation.

J. Curtis Nickel, MD
Department of Urology
Queen's University
Kingston, Ontario, Canada

E-mail address: jcn@queensu.ca

ELSEVIER
SAUNDERS

Urol Clin N Am 35 (2008) 1–12

UROLOGIC
CLINICS
of North America

Uncomplicated Urinary Tract Infection in Adults Including Uncomplicated Pyelonephritis

Lindsay E. Nicolle, MD, FRCPC

*Departments of Internal Medicine and Medical Microbiology, Health Sciences Centre, University of Manitoba,
Room GG443 – 820 Sherbrook Street, Winnipeg, MB R3A 1R9, Canada*

Acute uncomplicated urinary tract infection, also called acute uncomplicated cystitis, is a bladder infection that occurs in women who have normal structure and function of the genitourinary tract [1,2]. These same women are at risk for acute nonobstructive pyelonephritis, also called acute uncomplicated pyelonephritis. Women who experience recurrent acute uncomplicated urinary infection at a younger age continue to be at risk for recurrent infection after menopause [3–5], suggesting the determinants of uncomplicated infection in younger women continue to contribute in older women. Similarly, acute cystitis occurring in diabetic women without long-term complications of their diabetes, such as neuropathy, may be considered uncomplicated infection and managed as such. Acute urinary infection occurs rarely in young men with a normal genitourinary tract. When it does occur, risk associations include men who have sex with men [6,7] or a sexual partner with vaginal colonization with *E. coli* [8]. Lack of circumcision may also be a risk, but this association is more controversial [9]. These infections are so infrequent, however, that urinary infections in men should always be managed as complicated urinary infection.

Acute uncomplicated urinary infection

Epidemiology

As many as 10% of women experience at least one episode of acute uncomplicated urinary infection in a year, and 60% have at least one episode during their lifetime [10]. The peak incidence of infection occurs in young, sexually active, women aged 18 to 24 years [1]. Recurrent episodes are experienced by as many as 5% of women at some time during their life [11]. In a primary care setting, 44% of women presenting with an infection experienced a second infection within 1 year [12]; 21% of college women with a first urinary infection had a second infection within 6 months [13].

Acute cystitis is benign from the perspective of long-term outcomes, but is associated with substantial disruption in a woman's life with each episode. College women reported an average of 6.1 symptom days and 2 to 4 restricted activity days with an episode of cystitis, and 1.2 work days lost [14]. In a recent Canadian study of subjects presenting to family physicians, 63% of women reported the infection had an impact on their usual activities, with a mean duration of 4.9 days of symptoms [15].

Pathogenesis

Host factors

A genetic association is supported by the observation that women who experience recurrent cystitis are more likely than those without infections to have first degree female relatives (mothers, sisters, daughters) who also experience recurrent urinary tract infection [11]. Nonsecretor status may explain some of this predisposition, especially in older women [3,11,16]. Other potential genetic associations are not yet fully characterized.

Behavioral practices are strongly correlated with infection in young women. From 75% to 90% of episodes of cystitis in young sexually

E-mail address: lnicolle@hsc.mb.ca

doi:10.1016/j.ucl.2007.09.004

active women are attributable to sexual intercourse, with the frequency of infection correlating with the frequency of intercourse [11,16]. It is unusual for young women who are not sexually active to experience uncomplicated urinary infection [11,14]. The use of a spermicide for birth control is also a major behavioral risk for infection. The frequency of spermicide use correlates with the frequency of recurrent infection, independent of intercourse frequency [11,16,17]. Other behaviors previously considered risk factors for urinary infection have not been confirmed in repeated epidemiologic studies [11,17,18]. These activities include the use of birth control pill or condoms, postcoital voiding, type of underwear used, personal hygiene after voiding or defecating, or taking a bath rather than shower.

Risk factors for uncomplicated urinary infection differ in postmenopausal women. In prospective studies sexual activity is not associated with recurrent infection [4,19]. The strongest and most consistent risk factor for postmenopausal women is a history of urinary infection at a younger age [3,4,19]. Other potential contributors include diabetes [4] and nonsecretor status [3]. Chronic incontinence is consistently associated with urinary infection in postmenopausal women [3,4,19]. However, incontinence suggests the presence of voiding abnormalities, and these women would be assumed to have functional abnormalities consistent with complicated urinary infection.

Microbiology

Acute uncomplicated urinary infection is primarily a disease caused by extraintestinal pathogenic *Escherichia coli*; this organism is isolated in 80% to 85% of episodes [1,2,20]. Organisms that are capable of colonization and subsequent infection are characterized by a restricted number of phylogenetic *E. coli* groups and diverse virulence factors [21,22]. There is considerable overlap in putative virulence factors among strains isolated from symptomatic or asymptomatic infection [23]. The most important virulence factor for establishing bladder infection is likely the type 1, mannose sensitive, fimbria, which attaches to receptors on uroepithelial cells [24]. Unique strains of uropathogenic *E. coli* circulate among members of households [25], and may be isolated from clonal outbreaks in a community or larger geographic area [26].

Staphylococcus saprophyticus is the second most common organism isolated, although only 5% to 10% of episodes are attributed to this organism. It is isolated virtually only in the setting of acute uncomplicated cystitis. The genome of this bacteria has recently been characterized, and genetic elements contributing to success as a uropathogen have been described. These include an adhesin, transport systems supporting growth in urine, and a urease [27]. Other organisms are isolated infrequently. Group B streptococcus has a predilection for pregnant or diabetic women. *Proteus mirabilis* is uncommon, but may be isolated somewhat more frequently in postmenopausal women [20].

Antimicrobial resistance

Antimicrobial susceptibility of *E. coli* evolves continuously in response to antimicrobial pressure [20,28,29]. Increasing resistance has compromised the efficacy of ampicillin, cephalosporins, and trimethoprim/sulfamethoxazole (TMP/SMX), and increasing resistance to fluoroquinolones is now being reported [20]. The expansion of extended spectrum beta lactamase (ESBL) producing *E. coli*, usually also resistant to TMP/SMX and fluoroquinolones, is a current concern [30]. Resistance in community isolates occurs through both clonal expansion, as described with a TMP/SMX resistant *E. coli* strain in the United States [26], and through emergence in multiple distinct strains secondary to horizontal gene transfer, as reported in a study of isolates from Canada and Europe [31]. Prior recent antimicrobial therapy is the most important determinant for isolation of a resistant organism [29]. Antimicrobial pressure is attributable not just to prior treatment of urinary infection, but also antimicrobial use for other indications, such as the widespread use of fluoroquinolones for respiratory tract infection, or antimicrobial use in animal husbandry [32].

Origin of infection

Development of acute uncomplicated urinary infection follows colonization of the vagina and the periurethral area by uropathogenic *E. coli*. Colonization is characterized by replacement of the H_2O_2 producing lactobacilli (which maintain an acid vaginal environment) with *E. coli* and other organisms [33]. Spermicide use [34] and recent antimicrobial therapy [35] may facilitate these changes in flora, explaining the association of these behaviors with infection.

Recent studies in mice have reported that *E. coli* can persist within bladder uroepithelial cells. Early in the course of infection *E. coli* are internalized into these cells, which are then sloughed as part of the healing process [36]. It has been proposed that organisms that may persist within uroepithelial cells in the bladder are a reservoir for recurrent infection. The relevance of these observations to human beings has not yet been determined.

Diagnosis

Clinical

Acute uncomplicated urinary infection has a characteristic clinical presentation. New onset frequency, dysuria, and urgency, together with the absence of vaginal discharge or pain, has a positive predictive value of 90% for acute cystitis [37]. Infection may also be associated with hematuria. For older women, new or increased incontinence is also a common symptom. The presentation is so characteristic that women with a history of recurrent infection are over 90% accurate in self-diagnosis of infection [38,39].

Laboratory

The microbiologic diagnosis of urinary tract infection requires quantitative isolation of a uropathogenic organism from an appropriately collected urine specimen. A quantitative count of greater than or equal to 10^5 colony forming units (CFU) per mL (greater than or equal to 10^8 CFU/L) was initially proposed as the diagnostic criteria, based on studies primarily performed in asymptomatic women or women presenting with pyelonephritis. However, 30% to 50% of women presenting with clinical symptoms consistent with acute cystitis have lower quantitative counts, usually 10^3 CFU/mL to 10^5 CFU/mL [1,2]. Thus, greater than or equal to 10^3 CFU/mL of a uropathogen is the accepted microbiologic diagnostic criteria for acute cystitis [40]. As many as 10% to 20% of symptomatic women have negative urine cultures, presumably because of organism counts below the threshold for laboratory isolation. The clinical response to treatment for these women is similar to that of women with positive urine cultures [41].

Given the predictable microbiology, the limitations in interpretation of the quantitative urine culture, the reliable clinical diagnosis, and the 24 to 48 hour delay in culture results, it is recommended that empiric treatment be initiated based on symptoms alone, without consistent collection of a pretherapy urine specimen [2,42]. A specimen should be obtained, however, for women with an atypical presentation, with early symptomatic

recurrence after therapy, or when pyelonephritis is a potential diagnosis.

Pyuria is virtually a universal accompaniment of women with acute uncomplicated cystitis [1,42]. Documentation of pyuria supports the diagnosis and may be useful for evaluation of women who present with atypical symptoms. However, routine measurement of pyuria is not consistently recommended or necessary for management [1,43]. The absence of pyuria does not exclude the diagnosis of urinary infection in women with consistent symptoms [1,44].

Treatment

Natural history

Placebo controlled clinical trials have characterized the natural history of untreated acute cystitis [45,46]. Among 277 women treated with placebo, 28% were free of symptoms at 1 week and 45% had negative cultures by 6 weeks [46]. In another study, 54% of women who received placebo were asymptomatic by 3 days, and 52% at 7 days [45]. These studies suggest about half of women will have spontaneous clinical and microbiologic resolution of infection within a few days or weeks. Despite this, antimicrobial treatment substantially shortens the duration of symptoms. The clinical cure at 3 days was 77% with nitrofurantoin therapy, compared with 54% with placebo, and at 7 days 88%, compared with 52% with placebo [45]. In a recent clinical trial, 54% of subjects reported symptom improvement by 6 hours after therapy, 87% by 24 hours, and 91% by 48 hours [47]. By the fourth day of effective treatment 72% of patients had symptom resolution, and by the tenth day, 84% [15].

Antibiotic selection

Many antimicrobial regimens are effective for treatment (Table 1). The most common antimicrobials used include nitrofurantoin, TMP/SMX or trimethoprim alone, fluoroquinolones, beta-lactam antimicrobials including amoxicillin, cephalosporins and pivmecillinam, and fosfomycin trometamol. The efficacy of different antimicrobials varies, particularly for shorter durations of therapy. Beta-lactam antimicrobials, including amoxicillin, amoxicillin/clavulanic acid, and cephalosporins, are consistently less effective than TMP/SMX or fluoroquinolones [48]. In addition, nitrofurantoin and fosfomycin/trometamol are 5% to 10% less effective than 3 days of TMP/SMX or fluoroquinolone [1,2,48].

Table 1

Antimicrobial regimens effective for treatment of acute uncomplicated urinary infection

Agent	Dose	Duration
Amoxicillin	500 mg tid	7 days
Amoxicillin/clavulanic acid	500 mg tid	7 days
Cephalosporins:		
Cephalexin	250 mg–500 mg qid	7 days
Cefuroxime axetil	500 mg bid	7 days
Cefixime	400 mg od	7 days
Cefpodoxime proxetil	100 mg bid	3 days
Fluoroquinolones:		
Norfloxacin	400 mg bid	3 days
Ciprofloxacin	250 mg–500 mg bid	3 days
Extended release	500 mg od	3 days
Ofloxacin	200 mg	3 days
Levofloxacin	250 mg–500 mg bid	3 days
Nitrofurantoin macrocrystal	50 mg–100 mg qid	7 days
Monohydrate/ macrocrystals	100 mg bid	7 days
Pivmecillinam	400 mg bid	3 days
	200 mg bid	7 days
Fosfomycin trometamol	3 g	Single dose
TMP/SMX	160/800 mg bid	3 days
Trimethoprim	200 mg bid	3 days

Antimicrobial susceptibility is, of course, an important determinant of efficacy. Higher failure rates are observed for infections with TMP/SMX-resistant organisms treated with TMP/SMX [49]. In European countries where trimethoprim alone is frequently used, resistant rates over 20% are associated with high failure rates with empiric trimethoprim therapy [50]. *E. coli* strains generally remain susceptible to fluoroquinolones. However, the expansion of ESBL producing *E. coli* in community-acquired infections may limit future use [30]. Optimal treatment of urinary infection caused by ESBL producing *E. coli* is not well defined. Nitrofurantoin and fosfomycin trometamol remain effective for most of these strains. Pivmecillinam and amoxicillin/clavulanic acid may also be effective for some of these strains [51], although clinical experience is limited.

Duration of therapy

The recommended duration of therapy for acute cystitis is 3 days when trimethoprim, TMP/SMX, or a fluoroquinolone (norfloxacin, ciprofloxacin, levofloxacin) is prescribed [48,52].

For nitrofurantoin, 7-days therapy is recommended. Fosfomycin/trometamol is marketed only as single dose therapy. Pivmecillinam is recommended for treatment of 3 or 7 days; other beta-lactam antimicrobials are usually given as 7-day regimens, if used. A recent meta-analysis concluded that the 3-day therapy regimens are as effective as longer courses for resolution of symptoms, but may be less effective for microbiologic resolution [53]. However, randomized, placebo controlled clinical trials support the equivalent efficacy and fewer adverse effects of the shorter duration of therapy.

A single dose is quite effective for selected antimicrobials in addition to fosfomycin trometamol [54]. Cure rates with TMP/SMX and fluoroquinolones are reported to be 80% to 95% with a single dose. However, reviews and meta-analyses consistently report single dose therapy is marginally less effective than 3 days for TMP/SMX or fluoroquinolones [54]. In addition, patient and physician acceptance of a single dose regimen is problematic, as symptoms persist for several days after treatment while inflammation in the bladder resolves. Gatifloxacin was recently marketed with an indication for single dose therapy [55]; however, this agent has now been removed from the market because of serum glucose abnormalities.

Systematic reviews have concluded that a 3-day duration of therapy is not as effective for older, as compared with younger women [48,53]. Postmenopausal women, however, have poorer outcomes with any duration of antimicrobial therapy compared with premenopausal women [41]. A recent randomized, placebo controlled, trial compared 3 to 7 days of ciprofloxacin for acute cystitis in older women without complicating factors. The mean age of study participants was 78.5 years. Clinical and microbiologic outcomes were similar with either treatment duration, while 3 days of therapy was associated with significantly fewer adverse effects [56]. Thus, 3 days of therapy is appropriate for treatment of postmenopausal women with presumed uncomplicated infection.

Guidelines

Current guideline recommendations are summarized in Table 2. The Infectious Diseases Society of America (IDSA) guidelines, published in 1999, recommend TMP/SMX for 3 days as a first line treatment for acute uncomplicated cystitis [48]. However, if the prevalence of resistance of *E. coli* to TMP/SMX for isolates from acute uncomplicated cystitis in a region is over 20%,

Table 2
Recommendations of current guideline for treatment of acute uncomplicated urinary infection

IDSA	European Union
First line	
TMP/SMX, 3 days	TMP/SMX, 3 days
Alternatives	
Trimethoprim, 3 days	Cefpodoxime proxetil, 3 days
Fluoroquinolone (ofloxacin, norfloxacin, ciprofloxacin), 3 days	Ciprofloxacin, 3 days
	Fosfomycin trometamol, single dose
	Levofloxacin, 3 days
	Norfloxacin, 3 days
	Ofloxacin, 3 days
	Pivmecillinam, 7 days
	Trimethoprim, 5–7 days
Others	
Fosfomycin trometamol, single dose	Nitrofurantoin, 5–7 days
Nitrofurantoin, 7 days	Pivmecillinam, 3 days
	Trimethoprim, 3 days

an alternate antimicrobial should be selected for empiric treatment: nitrofurantoin for 7 days or one of the fluoroquinolones (norfloxacin, ciprofloxacin, levofloxacin) for 3 days would be recommended. The European Union guideline for acute uncomplicated cystitis was updated in 2006 [52]. This document also concludes that TMP/SMX for 3 days should be first line therapy, but emphasizes that knowledge of local resistance prevalence is essential in choosing empiric therapy. Effective alternate regimens for treatment of acute uncomplicated urinary infection are also recommended.

Managing recurrent infection

Delivery of care

Several management strategies have been described which allow prompt and efficient access to treatment for women with recurrent infection, while limiting costs. Effective approaches include telephone assessment and treatment by a physician [57] or nurse practitioner following an algorithm [43], or use of an interactive computer by the patient [58]. The general features of these strategies include no urine specimen collection, phone prescription without in-person assessment, and follow-up only if symptoms persist or recur early following treatment [42]. These approaches have been documented to be efficient, with increased patient satisfaction and cost savings, while treatment outcomes are equivalent to standard management by physician visit [43,57,58]. However, the studies were undertaken in relatively controlled settings with appropriate resources to support the program. The extent to which they are generally applicable may require evaluation in more diverse settings.

Self-treatment

Self-treatment by women who experience recurrent infection is also an effective strategy [38,39]. This approach may be particularly useful for women with infrequent recurrences, or who are concerned they may develop infection while traveling or otherwise unable to access usual health care. Women with recurrent urinary infection are over 90% accurate in identifying a new episode, and self-treatment is effective at least 85% of the time. Both single dose or 3 days of self-treatment with TMP/SMX or a fluoroquinolone have been shown to be effective, although current recommendations would be for a 3-day course. Women should be advised that failure of symptom resolution with treatment, or early recurrence following therapy, requires physician assessment.

Prevention

The first consideration in prevention is to address modifiable behavioral practices, particularly discontinuing the use of spermicide. Other effective strategies are generally considered as antimicrobial or nonantimicrobial (Table 3).

Low dose antimicrobial therapy remains an effective intervention to manage frequent, recurrent, acute uncomplicated urinary tract infection [1]. The antimicrobial may be given as continuous daily or every-other-day therapy, usually at bedtime, or as postcoital prophylaxis. First line treatments are nitrofurantoin or TMP/SMX. Fluoroquinolone antimicrobials are effective, but should be reserved for women who are unable to tolerate first line agents or who experience recurrent infection with resistant organisms while receiving first line regimens. The initial suggested duration of prophylaxis is 6 months; however, 50% of women will experience recurrence by 3 months after discontinuation of the prophylactic antimicrobial. When this occurs, prophylaxis may be reinstituted for as long as 1 or 2 years and remain effective.

Table 3
Strategies for prevention of recurrent acute uncomplicated urinary infection

Strategy	Efficacy
Long-term low dose antimicrobial prophylaxis	
• TMP/SMX 40/200 mg (1/2 regular strength) daily or eod	95%
• TMP 100 mg daily	95%
• Nitrofurantoin 50 mg or macrocrystals 100 mg daily	95%
• Norfloxacin 200 mg daily or eod	95%–100%
• Ciprofloxacin 125 mg daily	>95%
• Cephalexin 250 mg–500 mg daily	95%
Postcoital antimicrobial prophylaxis	
• Cephalexin 250 mg	>95%
• TMP/SMX 40/200 mg or 80/400 mg	90%–95%
• Trimethoprim 100 mg	>95%
• Nitrofurantoin 50 mg or 100 mg	>95%
• Norfloxacin 200 mg	>95%
• Ciprofloxacin 125 mg	>95%
Nonantimicrobial strategies	
• Cranberry or lingonberry juice or other products	20%–30%
• Probiotics	investigational
• Vaccination	investigational
• Topical estrogen for postmenopausal infections	0%–30%

Nonantimicrobial strategies to prevent recurrent infection are being developed and evaluated (see Table 3) [59]. Daily cranberry products (juice or tablets) or lingonberry juice decreases the frequency of recurrent infection by about 30%, compared with 90% to 95% effectiveness of antimicrobial use [60,61]. Vaccination strategies, and probiotics to re-establish vaginal colonization with H_2O_2 producing lactobacilli, are also being investigated, but studies to date do not report convincing efficacy [61,62]. Topical vaginal estrogen is a potential intervention to decrease recurrent episodes for postmenopausal women, but also remains controversial [63–67]. This approach may benefit some women, but is not as effective as antimicrobial prophylaxis. Systemic estrogen therapy is consistently associated with no benefit or an increased risk for infection [5,68].

Acute nonobstructive pyelonephritis

Acute nonobstructive pyelonephritis occurs in the same women who experience acute uncomplicated cystitis, but is less common. The relative frequency of pyelonephritis to cystitis for women with recurrent acute uncomplicated urinary infection was 18 to 1 [67] in a Seattle urinary infection referral cohort, and 29 to 1 in a Finland primary care cohort [12]. The genetic and behavioral risk factors associated with pyelonephritis are similar to those for acute, uncomplicated infection [68]. For premenopausal women, these include sexual intercourse, prior urinary infection, new sexual partner, recent spermicide use, urinary infection history in the mother, diabetes, and recent incontinence. The strongest association is with sexual intercourse. A recent study reports a familial susceptibility to pyelonephritis that may be attributable to low expression of CXCR1, an interleukin (IL)-8 receptor [69].

Pathogenesis

Microbiology

E. coli are isolated from about 90% of episodes of acute nonobstructive pyelonephritis. These pyelonephritogenic strains have unique virulence characteristics. The most consistent virulence factor is the presence of the P pilus, a Gal (∞ 1–4), Gal-β disaccharide galabiose adhesin [23]. There are several other virulence factors described, including hemolysin and Aerobactin. Virulence characteristics may cluster in pathogenic islands in the genome of uropathogenic strains.

The specific mechanisms by which E. coli produce pyelonephritis are not fully understood. In a normal urinary tract without reflux, virulence characteristics of infecting organisms must facilitate ascension from the bladder to the kidney, and subsequent adherence to renal cells in the medulla. Lipopolysaccharides released from the cell wall are thought to trigger an inflammatory response, which produces the clinical manifestations of illness.

Immune and inflammatory response

Pyelonephritis is characterized by the systemic and local production of cytokines and other inflammatory markers. These include proinflammatory cytokines, such as IL-6, IL-1 beta, and tumor necrosis factor (TNF)-alpha. IL-6 and IL-8 in serum and urine of patients are elevated in acute pyelonephritis [70], as are serum levels of granulocyte colony-stimulating factor (G-CSF) and IL-10 [71]. The IL-6 and G-CSF levels correlate with the presence of hemolysin and cytotoxic necrotizing factor in the infecting E. coli strain [70]. Serum levels of C-reactive protein, IL-6, and TNF-alpha are all elevated before antimicrobial therapy [72]. At 24 hours following initiation of antibiotics, the C-reactive protein and serum TNF-alpha remain elevated, as well as urinary N-acetyl-beta glucosaminidase, alpha-1 microglobulin, and beta-2 microglobulin. The serum IL-6 and urinary IL-6, IL-8, albumin, and immunoglobulin levels decrease significantly by 24 hours. The urine level of IL-8 at presentation and serum soluble IL-6 receptor level at 2 weeks may be prognostic markers for after-treatment recovery of the glomerular filtration rate [71]. The intensity of the inflammatory response in children with pyelonephritis correlates with development of renal scars and subsequent renal dysfunction, but this association has not yet been documented for adult women [72].

Diagnosis

Clinical

The clinical presentation of acute nonobstructive pyelonephritis is often straightforward, with signs and symptoms of costovertebral angle pain and tenderness, with or without fever, or lower tract irritative symptoms. However, the severity of symptoms at presentation is variable, with a spectrum ranging from predominantly lower tract symptoms with mild localizing costovertebral angle findings to severe systemic symptoms with bacteremia and sepsis. High fever, intense pain, and nausea and vomiting are common with severe presentations. The sepsis syndrome and septic shock are uncommon in women with acute uncomplicated pyelonephritis. Women presenting with more severe illness should always be considered, potentially, to have obstruction of the genitourinary tract rather than uncomplicated infection.

Urine culture

An appropriately collected urine specimen should always be obtained before the initiation of antimicrobial therapy. The quantitative count of greater than or equal to 10^4 CFU/mL, together with consistent symptoms of pyelonephritis, is considered diagnostic [40]. In addition to confirming the diagnosis, organism identification and antimicrobial susceptibility testing provides assurance that the initial empiric therapy is appropriate, and allows selection of a specific oral agent to complete therapy after an initial response to parenteral therapy.

Other laboratory tests

A complete blood count, blood urea, and creatinine should be obtained. The leukocyte count is a measure of disease severity, and can be monitored as an indicator of infection resolution and response to therapy. Renal failure is unusual with uncomplicated pyelonephritis, but acute or chronic renal impairment must always be excluded.

When blood cultures were obtained uniformly from all women with uncomplicated pyelonephritis presenting to a Spanish hospital, 25.2% were positive [73]. For women or children admitted to an American hospital with uncomplicated pyelonephritis, 50% had blood cultures obtained and 10.4% of these were bacteremic [74]. Positive blood cultures were concordant with urine cultures in over 95% of cases, and clinical outcomes did not differ for women with or without bacteremia [73,74]. Thus, obtaining routine blood cultures for all patients with pyelonephritis does not have clinical utility. However, any women with presentations including high fever, hemodynamic instability, or severe nausea and vomiting, or in whom the diagnosis is uncertain, should have blood cultures obtained.

C-reactive protein and procalcitonin levels are elevated with acute pyelonephritis [75,76]. The measurement of levels of these proteins as diagnostic tests or prognostic indicators has been studied in pediatric populations. It is not clear whether the tests are useful in management of women with nonobstructive pyelonephritis. In one study, serum procalcitonin level at presentation did not predict a poor outcome [75].

Diagnostic imaging

It has been suggested that all women presenting with acute pyelonephritis require imaging of the genitourinary tract [77,78]. Ultrasound studies are used most frequently, but are relatively insensitive. They usually show enlargement of one or both affected kidneys, with focal complications identified in less than 10% [79]. Computerized tomography (CT) may be the imaging modality of choice. It will identify calculi, gas, hemorrhage, calcification, obstruction, renal enlargement, and inflammatory masses. Contrast enhanced scans are recommended; helical and multislice CT allow study of different phases of contrast excretion [80]. It is not clear, however, that routine imaging for all subjects has utility in management of infection or leads to improved outcomes [78]. Diagnostic imaging is useful when the diagnosis is uncertain, with more severe presentations when obstruction or abscess must be expeditiously excluded, or if there is inadequate response or rapid recurrence following appropriate therapy and an underlying abnormality must be excluded [80]. On the other hand, a woman presenting with mild or moderate symptoms, who responds promptly to antimicrobial therapy with no recurrence, is unlikely to benefit from imaging studies. Thus, diagnostic imaging should be used selectively.

Management

Hospitalization

The initial assessment of any woman presenting with acute nonobstructive pyelonephritis includes evaluation of the severity of illness. Temperature, blood pressure, and symptoms such as vomiting should be noted. The majority, probably 80%, of young women with acute pyelonephritis do not require hospitalization and are effectively treated with oral therapy, often with an initial intravenous dose of antimicrobials. Women should be considered for hospitalization and initial parenteral therapy if they are hemodynamically unstable, have severe nausea and vomiting, or if there are concerns about absorption of oral antimicrobials. Appropriate supportive management for hypotension, vomiting, and pain control should be initiated promptly.

Antimicrobial treatment

Antimicrobial levels achieved in renal tissue are generally similar to plasma concentrations, rather than the high levels achieved in renal tubules and urine. Aminoglycosides may have a unique role for treatment of pyelonephritis, as they are reabsorbed and bound in the proximal tubular epithelium, leading to higher concentrations in renal tissue than in plasma [81]. There are few comparative clinical trials addressing treatment of acute uncomplicated pyelonephritis [48,52]. Despite this, several antimicrobial regimens are clearly effective (Box 1). The selection of empiric therapy is based on patient tolerance, history of prior antimicrobial therapy, and suspected or known local prevalence of resistance to *E. coli*.

For first line parenteral therapy, a fluoroquinolone with renal excretion, a second or third generation cephalosporin, an aminopenicillin with a beta lactamase inhibitor, or an aminoglycoside with or without ampicillin are recommended (Table 4) [48,52]. When an ESBL producing *E. coli* is suspected, optimal initial empiric parenteral therapy may be ertapenem, although there is limited clinical experience to date. Initial parenteral therapy should be reviewed after

---

Box 1. Antimicrobial regimens of documented efficacy for management of acute uncomplicated pyelonephritis

Parenteral regimens
Aminoglycoside (gentamicin or tobramycin 3 mg/kg–5 mg/kg once daily in 1–3 doses)
   +/− ampicillin 1–2 g every 4 hours
TMP/SMX 160/800 mg twice a day
Ciprofloxacin 400 mg twice a day
Ceftriaxone 1 g intravenously every 24 hours
Cefotaxime 1 g intravenously every 8 hours

Oral regimens
Cefpodoxime proxetil 200 mg twice a day for 10 days
Ciprofloxacin 500 mg twice a day for 7 days
   Extended release 1 g once daily for 7 to 10 days
Levofloxacin 250 mg once a day for 10 days
Lomefloxacin 400 mg once a day for 10 days
TMP/SMX 160/800 mg twice a day for 14 days

---

48 to 72 hours to assess the clinical response and review urine culture results. In most cases, the antimicrobial course can then be completed with oral therapy.

Patients with less severe presentations may be started initially on empiric oral therapy or given an initial single parenteral dose of a fluoroquinolone, aminoglycoside, or ceftriaxone, then oral therapy (see Table 4). Generally an oral fluoroquinolone—ciprofloxacin or levofloxacin—is recommended. If the organism is susceptible, TMP/SMX is an alternate effective treatment. Optimal oral therapy for treatment of pyelonephritis with ESBL producing *E. coli* is not yet determined.

Duration of treatment and follow-up

The recommended duration of antibiotic therapy is generally 10 to 14 days. A 7-day course of treatment is also effective, at least for fluoroquinolones [52,82]. Older studies enrolling small numbers of subjects reported successful outcome

Table 4
Current guideline recommendations for treatment of acute, uncomplicated pyelonephritis

IDSA	European Union
Oral	
First line	*First line*
Fluoroquinolone, 7–14 days (ciprofloxacin, levofloxacin)	Fluoroquinolone, 7 days
Alternates	*Alternates*
TMP/SMX, 14 days (if susceptible)	Aminopenicillin plus beta-lactamase inhibitor
Amoxicillin (for Gram positive)	Cephalosporin (third generation)
Amoxicillin/clavulanic acid (for Gram positive)	TMP/SMX (if susceptible)
Parenteral	
Aminoglycoside plus or minus ampicillin	Fluoroquinolone
Fluoroquinolone	Aminopenicillin/ β-lactamase inhibitor
Extended spectrum cephalosporin	Third generation cephalosporin
	Aminoglycoside

with treatment courses of only 5 days of gentamicin, but these very short durations have not been confirmed in clinical trials and cannot currently be recommended.

The majority of women will be afebrile by 48 to 72 hours after initiation of effective antimicrobial therapy. Risk factors for a poor outcome include hospitalization, isolation of a resistant organism, concurrent diabetes mellitus, and a history of renal stones [83]. Repeat urine cultures during follow-up are not recommended for women who remain asymptomatic.

Summary

Acute uncomplicated urinary tract infection and acute pyelonephritis are common infections that occur in a substantial number of otherwise healthy women. The treatment of individual episodes is generally straightforward, with the more difficult management problem being the effective treatment and prevention of recurrent infection. There is substantial knowledge describing precipitating factors for infection, particularly the pivotal role of sexual intercourse. However, further investigation to more fully characterize genetic associations is needed. The evolution of antimicrobial susceptibility in community-acquired *E. coli* requires continued reassessment of optimal empiric antimicrobial therapy for both cystitis and pyelonephritis.

References

[1] Fihn SD. Acute uncomplicated urinary tract infection in women. N Engl J Med 2003;349:259–66.

[2] Hooton TM. The current management strategies for community-acquired urinary tract infection. Infect Dis Clin North Am 2003;17:303–22.

[3] Raz R, Gennesin Y, Wasser J, et al. Recurrent urinary tract infections in postmenopausal women. Clin Infect Dis 2000;30:152–6.

[4] Hu KK, Boyko EJ, Scholes D, et al. Risk factors for urinary tract infections in postmenopausal women. Arch Intern Med 2004;164:989–93.

[5] Jackson SL, Boyko EJ, Scholes D, et al. Predictor of urinary tract infection after menopause: a prospective study. Am J Med 2004;117:903–11.

[6] Barnes RC, Daifuku R, Roddy RE, et al. Urinary tract infection in sexually active homosexual men. Lancet 1986;25:171–3.

[7] Russell DB, Roth NJ. Urinary tract infections in men in a primary care population. Aust Fam Physician 2001;30:177–9.

[8] Foxman B, Manning SD, Tallman P, et al. Uropathogenic *Escherichia coli* are more likely than commensal *E. coli* to be shared between heterosexual sex partners. Am J Epidemiol 2002;156:1133–40.

[9] Spach DH, Stapleton AE, Stamm WE. Lack of circumcision increases the risk of urinary tract infection in young men. JAMA 1992;267:679–81.

[10] Foxman B, Barlow R, D'Arcy H, et al. Urinary tract infection: self-reported incidence and associated costs. Ann Epidemiol 2000;10:509–15.

[11] Scholes D, Hooton TM, Roberts PL, et al. Risk factors for recurrent urinary tract infection in young women. J Infect Dis 2000;182:1177–82.

[12] Ikaheimo R, Siitonen A, Heiskanen T, et al. Recurrence of urinary tract infection in a primary care setting: analysis of a one-year follow-up of 179 women. Clin Infect Dis 1996;22:91–9.

[13] Foxman B, Gillespie B, Koopman J, et al. Risk factors for second urinary tract infection among college women. Am J Epidemiol 2000;151:1194–205.

[14] Foxman B, Frerichs RR. Epidemiology of urinary tract infection: diaphragm use and sexual intercourse. Am J Public Health 1985;75:1308–13.

[15] Nickel JC, Lee JC, Grantmyre JE, et al. Natural history of urinary tract infection in a primary care environment in Canada. Can J Urol 2005;12:2718–37.

[16] Hooton TM, Scholes D, Hughes JP, et al. A prospective study of risk factors for symptomatic urinary infection in young women. N Engl J Med 1996;335:468–74.

[17] Foxman B, Fricks RR. Epidemiology of urinary tract infection: II. Diet, clothing, and urination habits. Am J Public Health 1985;75:1314–7.

[18] Remis RS, Gurwith MJ, Gurwith D, et al. Risk factors for urinary tract infection. Am J Epidemiol 1987;126:685–94.

[19] Foxman B, Somsel P, Tallman P, et al. Urinary tract infection among women aged 40 to 65: behavioral and sexual risk factors. J Clin Epidemiol 2001;54:710–8.

[20] Kahlmeter G. ECO.SENS. An international survey of the antimicrobial susceptibility of pathogens from uncomplicated urinary tract infections: the ECO.SENS project. J Antimicrob Chemother 2003;51:69–76.

[21] Johnson JR, Owens K, Gajewski A, et al. Bacterial characteristics in relation to clinical source of Escherichia coli isolates from women with acute cystitis or pyelonephritis and uninfected women. J Clin Microbiol 2005;43:6064–72.

[22] Johnson JR. Microbial virulence determinants and the pathogenesis of urinary tract infection. Infect Dis Clin North Am 2003;17:261–78.

[23] Takahashi A, Kanamaru S, Kurazono H, et al. Escherichia coli isolates associated with uncomplicated and complicated cystitis and asymptomatic bacteriuria possess similar phylogenies, virulence genes, and O-serogroup profiles. J Clin Microbiol 2006;44:4589–92.

[24] Gunther NW, Lockatell J, Johnson DE, et al. In vivo dynamics of type 1 fimbria regulation in uropathogenic Escherichia coli during experimental urinary tract infection. Infect Immun 2001;69:2838–46.

[25] Johnson JR, Clabots C. Sharing of virulent Escherichia coli clones among household members of a woman with acute cystitis. Clin Infect Dis 2006; 43:c101–8.

[26] Manges AR, Johnson JR, Foxman B, et al. Widespread distribution of urinary tract infections caused by a multidrug-resistant Escherichia coli clonal group. N Engl J Med 2001;345:1007–13.

[27] Kuroda M, Yamashita A, Hirakawa H, et al. Whole genome sequence of Staphylococcus saprophyticus reveals the pathogenesis of uncomplicated urinary tract infection. Proc Natl Acad Sci U S A 2005; 102:12372–3277.

[28] Gupta K, Sahm DF, Mayfield D, et al. Antimicrobial resistance among uropathogens that cause community-acquired urinary tract infections in women: a nationwide analysis. Clin Infect Dis 2001;33: 89–94.

[29] Gupta K. Addressing antibiotic resistance. Am J Med 2002;113(1A):29S–34S.

[30] Pitout JD, Gregson DB, Church PL, et al. Community-wide outbreaks of clonally related CTX-M-14 beta-lactamase-producing Escherichia coli strains in the Calgary health region. J Clin Microbiol 2005;43:2844–9.

[31] Blahna MT, Zalewski CA, Reuer J, et al. The role of horizontal gene transfer in the spread of trimethoprim-sulfamethoxazole resistance among uropathogenic Escherichia coli in Europe and Canada. J Antimicrob Chemother 2006;57:666–72.

[32] Ramchandani M, Manges AR, DebRoy C, et al. Possible animal origin of human-associated, multidrug-resistant, uropathogenic Escherichia coli. Clin Infect Dis 2005;40:251–7.

[33] Gupta K, Stapleton AE, Hooton TM, et al. Inverse association of H_2O_2-producing lactobacilli and vaginal Escherichia coli colonization in women with recurrent urinary tract infection. J Infect Dis 1998;178: 446–50.

[34] Gupta K, Hillier SL, Hooton TM, et al. Effects of contraceptive method on the vaginal microbial flora: a prospective evaluation. J Infect Dis 2000;181: 595–601.

[35] Smith HS, Hughes JP, Hooton TM, et al. Antecedent antimicrobial use increases the risk of uncomplicated cystitis in young women. Clin Infect Dis 1997; 25:63–8.

[36] Garofalo CK, Hooton TM, Martin SM, et al. Escherichia coli from urine of female patients with urinary tract infections is competent for intracellular bacterial community formation. Infect Immun 2007; 75:52–60.

[37] Bent S, Nallamothu BK, Simel DL, et al. Does this women have an acute uncomplicated urinary tract infection? JAMA 2002;287:2701–10.

[38] Schaeffer AJ, Stuppy BA. Efficacy and safety of self-start therapy in women with recurrent urinary tract infections. J Urol 1999;161:207–11.

[39] Gupta K, Hooton TM, Roberts PL, et al. Patient-initiated treatment of uncomplicated recurrent urinary tract infections in young women. Ann Intern Med 2001;135:9–16.

[40] Rubin RH, Shapiro ED, Andriole VT, et al. Evaluation of new anti-infective drugs for the treatment of urinary tract infection. Clin Infect Dis 1992;15:S216–27.

[41] Nicolle LE, Madsen KS, Debeeck GD, et al. Three days of pivmecillinam or norfloxacin for treatment of acute uncomplicated urinary infection in women. Scand J Infect Dis 2002;34:487–92.

[42] Bent S, Saint S. The optimal use of diagnostic testing in women with acute uncomplicated cystitis. Am J Med 2002;113(Suppl 1A):20S–8S.

[43] Saint S, Scholes D, Fihn SD, et al. The effectiveness of a clinical practice guideline for the management of presumed uncomplicated urinary tract infection in women. Am J Med 1999;106:636–41.

[44] Nys S, van Merode T, Bartelds AIM, et al. Urinary tract infections in general practice patients: diagnostic tests versus bacteriological culture. J Antimicrob Chemother 2006;57:955–8.

[45] Christiaens TC, DeMeyere M, Versctiraegen G, et al. Randomized controlled trial of nitrofurantoin versus placebo in the treatment of uncomplicated urinary tract infection in adult women. Br J Gen Pract 2002;52:729–34.

[46] Ferry SA, Holm LSE, Stenlund H, et al. The natural course of uncomplicated lower urinary tract infection in women illustrated by a randomized controlled study. Scand J Infect Dis 2004;36:296–301.

[47] Klimberg I, Shockey G, Ellison H, et al. Time to symptom relief for uncomplicated urinary tract infection treated with extended release ciprofloxacin: a prospective, open-label, uncontrolled primary care study. Curr Med Res Opin 2005;21:1241–50.

[48] Warren JW, Abrutyn E, Hebel JR, et al. Guidelines for antimicrobial treatment of uncomplicated acute bacterial cystitis and acute pyelonephritis in women. Clin Infect Dis 1999;29:745–58.

[49] Raz R, Chazan B, Kennes Y, et al. Empiric use of trimethoprim-sulfamethoxazole in the treatment of women with uncomplicated urinary tract infections in a geographical area with a high prevalence of TMP-SMX resistant organisms. Clin Infect Dis 2002;34:1165–9.

[50] McNulty CAM, Richards J, Livermore DM, et al. Clinical relevance of laboratory-reported antibiotic resistance in acute uncomplicated urinary tract infection in primary care. J Antimicrob Chemother 2006;58:1000–8.

[51] Thomas K, Weinbren MJ, Warner M, et al. Activity of mecillinam against ESBL producers in vitro. J Antimicrob Chemother 2006;57:367–8.

[52] Naber KG, Bishop MC, Bjerklund-Johansen TE, et al. Guidelines on the management of urinary and male genital tract infections. Ipp 1–126: European Association of Urology: Guidelines. 2007 edition. ISBN-13:978-90-70244-59-D.

[53] Katchman EA, Milo G, Paul M, et al. Three day versus long duration of antibiotic treatment for cystitis in women: systematic review and meta-analysis. Am J Med 2005;118:1196–207.

[54] Nicolle LE. Short term therapy for urinary tract infection: Success and failure. Int J Antimicrob Chemother 2007; in press.

[55] Richard GA, Mathew CP, Kirstein JM, et al. Single dose fluoroquinolone therapy of acute uncomplicated urinary tract infection in women: results from a randomized, double-blind, multicenter trial comparing single-dose to 3-day fluoroquinolone regimens. Urology 2002;59:334–9.

[56] Vogel T, Verreault R, Gourdeau M, et al. Optimal duration of antibiotic therapy for uncomplicated urinary tract infection in older women: a double-blind randomized controlled trial. Can Med Assoc J 2004;170:469–73.

[57] Barry HC, Hickner J, Ebell MH, et al. A randomized, controlled trial of telephone management of suspected urinary tract infections in women. J Fam Pract 2001;50:589–94.

[58] Aagaard EM, Nadler P, Adler J, et al. An interactive computer kiosk module for the treatment of recurrent uncomplicated cystitis in women. J Gen Intern Med 2006;21:1156–9.

[59] Stapleton A. Novel approaches to prevention of urinary tract infections. Infect Dis Clin North Am 2003;17:457–71.

[60] Kontiokari T, Sundqvist K, Nuutinen M, et al. Randomized trial of cranberry lingonberry juice or Lactobacillus GG drink for the prevention of urinary tract infections in women. Br Med J 2001;322:1571.

[61] Stothers L. A randomized trial to evaluate effectiveness and cost-effectiveness of naturopathic cranberry products as prophylaxis against urinary tract infection. Can J Urol 2002;9:1558–62.

[62] Raz R, Stamm WE. A controlled trial of intravaginal estriol in postmenopausal women with recurrent urinary tract infections. N Engl J Med 1993;329:753–6.

[63] Erikson BC. A randomized, open, parallel group study on the preventive effect of an estradiol-releasing vaginal ring on recurrent urinary tract infections in postmenopausal women. Am J Obstet Gynecol 1999;180:1072–9.

[64] Cardozo L, Bennes C, Abbott D. Low dose oestrogen prophylaxis for recurrent urinary tract infections in elderly women. Br J Obstet Gynaecol 1998; 105:403–7.

[65] Raz R, Colodner R, Rohana Y, et al. Effectiveness of estriol-containing vaginal pessaries and nitrofurantoin macrocrystal therapy in the prevention of recurrent urinary tract infection in post-menopausal women. Clin Infect Dis 2003;36:1362–8.

[66] Brown JS, Vittinghoff E, Kanaya AM, et al. Urinary tract infections in postmenopausal women: effect of hormone therapy and risk factors. Obstet Gynecol 2001;98:1045–52.

[67] Stamm WE, McKevitt M, Roberts PL, et al. Natural history of recurrent urinary tract infections in women. Rev Infect Dis 1991;12:77–84.

[68] Scholes D, Hooton TM, Roberts PL, et al. Risk factors associated with acute pyelonephritis in healthy women. Ann Intern Med 2005;142:20–7.

[69] Lundstedt A-C, Leijonhufuad I, Ragnarsdottie B, et al. Inherited susceptibility to acute pyelonephritis: A family study of urinary tract infection. J Infect Dis 2007;195:1227–34.

[70] Jacobson SH, Hylander B, Wretlind B, et al. Interleukin-6 and interleukin-8 in serum and urine in patients with acute pyelonephritis in relation to bacterial-virulence-associated traits and renal function. Nephron 1994;67:172–9.

[71] Jacobson SH, Lu Y, Brauner A. Soluble interleukin-6 receptor, interleukin-10 and granulocyte colony-stimulating factor in acute pyelonephritis: relationship to markers of bacterial virulence and renal function. Nephron 1998;80:401–7.

[72] Horcajada JP, Valasco M, Filella X, et al. Evaluation of inflammatory and renal-injury markers in women treated with antibiotics for acute pyelonephritis caused by Escherichia coli. Clin Diagn Lab Immunol 2004;11:142–6.

[73] Velasco M, Martinez JA, Moreno-Martinez A, et al. Blood cultures for women with uncomplicated acute pyelonephritis: are they necessary? Clin Infect dis 2003;45:1127–30.

[74] Pasternak EL 3rd, Topinka MA. Blood cultures in pyelonephritis: do results change therapy? Acad Emerg Med 2000;7:1170.

[75] Lemiale V, Renaud B, Moutereau S, et al. A single procalcitonin level does not predict adverse outcomes of women with pyelonephritis. Eur Urol 2007;51:1394–401.

[76] Jellheden B, Norrby RS, Sandberg T. Symptomatic urinary tract infection in women in primary health care. Bacteriological, clinical and diagnostic aspects in relation to host response to infection. Scand J Prim Health Care 1996;14:122–8.

[77] Johnssen TE. The role of imaging in urinary tract infections. World J Urol 2004;22:392–8.

[78] Shen Y, Brown MA. Renal imaging in pyelonephritis. J Urol 2005;173:845–6.

[79] Johnson JR, Vincent LM, Wang K, et al. Renal ultrasonographic correlates of acute pyelonephritis. Clin Infect Dis 1992;14:15–22.

[80] Stunell H, Buckley O, Feeney J, et al. Imaging of acute pyelonephritis in the adult. Eur Radiol 2002; 17:1820–8.

[81] Frimodt-Moller N. Correlation between pharmaco-kinetic/pharmacodynamic parameters and efficacy for antibiotics in the treatment of urinary tract infection. Int J Antimicrob Agents 2002;19: 546–53.

[82] Talan DA, Stamm WE, Hooton TM, et al. Comparison of ciprofloxacin (7 days) and trimethoprim-sulfamethoxazole (14 days) for acute uncomplicated pyelonephritis in women. J Am Med Assoc 2000; 283:1583–90.

[83] Pertel PE, Haverstock D. Risk factors for a poor outcome after therapy for acute pyelonephritis. Brit J Urol Int 2006;98:141–7.

**ELSEVIER
SAUNDERS**

Urol Clin N Am 35 (2008) 13–22

**UROLOGIC
CLINICS
of North America**

Complicated Urinary Tract Infections

Durwood E. Neal, Jr, MD

*Division of Urology, Department of Surgery, M562,
#1 Hospital Drive – DOC80.00, University of Missouri, Columbia, MO 65212, USA*

The definition of complicated versus uncomplicated urinary tract infection (UTI) is one of practicality and necessity, and as such, it accomplishes several goals. First, complicated UTI describes a group of patients that usually need a prolonged course of antimicrobial therapy, with all its attendant morbidities, costs, and outcome differences. Second, it selects patients who may need interventional therapeutics, including surgery, endoscopy, or other modalities. Third, it follows that the patients denoted by this definition will most likely need to be managed, at least to some extent, by a trained urologic surgeon. With that prologue, a definition of complicated urinary tract infection must define the patient population, clinical conditions, and minimum necessary evaluation. A complicated urinary tract infection is that which occurs in a patient with an anatomically abnormal urinary tract or significant medical or surgical comorbidities [1]. Whereas this definition may not cover each and every situation, it does serve to encompass the great majority of these patients and guide their care. Both parts are necessarily broad, to assure that these potentially complex patients are appropriately managed.

There are a number of characteristics that may serve to describe complicated UTIs (Box 1). The first is that they, like uncomplicated UTIs, are almost always ascending in nature [2,3]. The periurethral tissues become colonized and the urethra eventually becomes involved. From there, the bladder in a female is colonized, or the prostate in a male. The organism, once it reaches the bladder, usually has little difficulty in establishing a stronghold and either invading or further

ascending, or both. There are a few exceptions to this rule, renal infection in intravenous drug abuse among them. The most common organisms in this scenario are the skin flora, more specifically, *Staphylococcus aureus*. A second exception consists of patients with miliary infections that start elsewhere, at another point of entry, and then are hematogenously transported to the kidneys. Because the blood supply is so exuberant, a common sequela is renal. The prototypical infection of this type is *Mycobacterium tuberculosis*, but others may cause this as well from varied sources, spanning the common bacteria to the fungi and fastidious microorganisms. In the incipience, *Escherichia coli* tends to be the first infection in many cases [3], but subsequent infections may be anything, often with a varying resistance by antibiogram. Polymicrobial infections are the exception rather than the rule, and most of the time there is a solitary microbe. A notable exception to this is in patients with a chronic indwelling catheter, because they may have a number of organisms present by culture. The challenge in this circumstance is to discern which organism is the one that is actually causing the infection.

Because defining which antimicrobials are of the utmost importance, the clinician must often use the broadest spectrum of drugs, or even multiples. With this in mind, there is often a wider array of pathogens that may be operative in complicated UTIs [4]. This is a result of several factors. This first of these is location of patient exposure. Nosocomial infections, by the sheer volume of susceptible individuals and variety of organisms present, are common [5]. A second reason is that because many more of those microorganisms may have access to the patient and persistence is common, there may be more varied

---

E-mail address: nealde@health.missouri.edu

> **Box 1. Characteristics of complicated UTI**
>
> 1. Usually ascending
> 2. Defined susceptible population
> 3. Drug resistance common
> 4. Prolonged therapy

> **Box 2. Complicating factors**
>
> Indwelling catheters
> Obstruction
> Male gender
> Age
> Diabetes mellitus
> Renal insufficiency
> Immunosuppression
> Urolithiasis
> Surgery
> Voiding dysfunction
> Valves
> Reflux
> Pregnancy
> Nosocomial

etiologic agents. A third is that because some of these microbes have a limited ability to infect immunologically sound patients, and by definition some of the patients included in the category of complicated UTIs have compromised immune systems, they may have greater access to hosts. Drug resistance tends to be more common in patients with complicated UTIs [6–8], which may be caused by exposure to more antibiotics, and thus the selective process may have a major role. The place of acquisition of the infection must be factored in also, as accessibility to susceptible host is a key contribution. Because bacteria are known to exchange DNA with one another, using the analogy of sexually transmitted diseases, more organisms may gain resistance, thus acquiring a survival advantage. Hospitals and nursing homes are the places where these circumstances abound [9].

Host factors: which patients are at risk for complicated UTI

Intubated urinary tract

The patient with an intubated urinary tract, whether it is an indwelling catheter (urethral, suprapubic, nephrostomy, or others) or an internal one, such as a ureteral or urethral, would always be included in this group of patients at risk for complicated UTI (Box 2) [10,11]. The first reason for this is that they are always at increased risk for infection and, with subsequent exposure to multiple courses of antibiotics, prone to infections with resistant organisms. The second reason, at least at first examination, is that urinary findings of infection may be indistinguishable from those with sterile urine, from the perspective of the urinary chemistry (leukocyste esterase, nitrite, hemoglobin, and others), as well as the microscopy of the urinary sediment. It has been shown that in the presence of an indwelling catheter, the urine will become colonized, if not infected by the 2-week time period. Rarely is the urinary

tract sterile beyond this epoch. The usual organisms tend to be uropathogens, but occasionally skin flora or vaginal organisms predominate. Often it is difficult to distinguish colonization from frank infection in the setting of an indwelling catheter.

Urinary obstruction

The patient with a known urinary obstruction, whether it involves the upper or lower urinary tract, must be similarly included [4], even if it is a patient who has had prior treatment for their obstruction. It should be assumed that even a corrected obstruction might not have rendered the problem completely resolved. Obstruction allows for the prolongation of bacteriuria by mechanical means, but also interferes with the local and systemic immune response, preventing its functioning at optimal levels. Lastly, the bacteria themselves are capable of effectively altering their microenvironment, which allows for prolongation of bacterial survival, improved colonization, and growth enhancement. There are a number of mechanisms by which this is accomplished and will be covered later in this article. The infectious process in and of itself increases the degree of obstruction. This is accomplished by bacterial alterations of the environment in the course of the infection, resulting in swelling and prevention of peristalsis [12]. In addition, there are a number of products produced by the bacteria that paralyze the urinary tract. The presence of obstruction causes the kidney to have a reduced ability to excrete and concentrate antibiotics as well, and may reduce the ability of the drug to function because of the extended presence of bacterial products in the environment. In the setting of obstruction, an infection may be viewed as an undrained abscess. This would naturally depend upon the degree of obstruction and also the level of the urinary tract where the obstruction has occurred. In most cases, however, drainage is indicated, usually on an urgent or even emergent basis.

Male gender

Most clinicians would suggest that male gender alone is criteria for being a complicated UTI [1,13]. This would be especially true in the mature individual who likely would have some element of benign prostatic hyperplasia, and thus presumably a lower urinary tract obstruction [14]. It could be postulated that because males have several advantages over females when it comes to urinary tract infection susceptibility, an infection in this gender should raise suspicion of an underlying condition. The presence of an elongated urethra (enhanced mechanical barrier) and the antibacterial nature of prostatic secretions combine to reduce the incidence of UTIs in this group as a whole [15]. Thus, infection in a male suggests mitigating influences, causing a condition where these enhanced defuse symptoms have been a complicated situation. Knowing that infection of the prostate gland can require a longer course of therapy further solidifies these patients in the complicated category.

Age

Age is always a consideration when considering the existence of a complicated UTI. Infections in childhood portend certain abnormalities of the genitourinary tract [16,17]. Vesicoureteral reflux, urethral valves, ureteropelvic obstruction, or ureterovesical obstruction are all relatively common conditions where there is a penchant for an increased incidence of urinary tract infections, as well as increased severity. What is more, UTIs in adults may be, at least in part, caused by behavioral circumstances such as sexual activity, which are less likely scenarios in the child. Gender here is important as well, in that, for the most part, congenital genitourinary abnormalities are more common in boys than girls. When discussing UTIs in children, the subject always surfaces regarding the role of circumcision. It is clear that circumcised boys rarely have UTIs, but that routine prophylactic circumcision to avoid UTIs is

not indicated. There are instances in which circumcision may be indicated for boys with certain congenital urologic conditions, in whom UTIs are more ominous, and therefore circumcision is indicated from a preventative prospective [18].

Diabetes

A number of medical conditions have been shown to be risk factors for UTIs, and moreover, lead to a more protracted course of therapy with potentially adverse outcomes because of specific complications. One of the most important of these is diabetes mellitus (DM). Not only are these patients more susceptible to UTIs in general, but also some of the complications are observed far more often in these patients [19–21]. Perinephric abscesses are rarely seen in patients without obstruction, except in the setting of diabetes, particularly when there is poor glucose control. This is also true for lobar nephronia, intrarenal abscesses, or carbuncles. One condition that is almost exclusive to diabetics is emphysematous pyelonephritis [22]. This is a specific case of renal infection that is manifested by the presence of gas in the renal parenchyma. The condition has a mortality rate that exceeds 40% and often results in loss of the affected kidney. Secondary obstruction may also be seen in DM because of the sloughing of papillae. This results in obstruction of the upper urinary tract by mechanical means. The pathophysiology is a result of pyelonephritis in a patient with compromised intrarenal blood flow, as is often the case with diabetics. This, then, presents an emergency requiring immediate drainage by either a retrograde or antegrade technique. Lastly, patients with DM have a strong predilection for having asymptomatic bacteriuria. This always presents the clinician with a dilemma as to whether to treat the patient with antibiotics or not. No good data as to the management exists, but if a patient has a history of febrile UTIs or any other comorbidity, the risk inherent in nontreatment is unacceptably high [23].

Renal insufficiency

Patients with renal insufficiency are another high-risk group, and must be included in the discussion of complicated UTIs [24,25]. The reason for this is because of the reduction in renal blood flow that most often accompanies this disease. The secondary effects of this include a reduced immune response, both on the local and systemic level. Depending on the degree of reduced renal function, there may also be a reduced urinary volume, which can impair host defenses and increase the bacterial capability to colonize the urinary tract. The changes that take place in the urine itself are that concentrating ability is reduced and the subsequent marshalling of substances inhibitory to bacterial growth are limited. Uremia itself impairs the immune system and may make it difficult to clear infections. In the end stages of renal failure, complicated UTIs increase, as does the morbidity. The delivery of antibiotics anywhere in the urinary tract, from the kidney to the urethra, is compromised, making eradication of infection a daunting proposition. That, coupled with the reduced immune response, makes the morbidity and mortality very high. When there is a bladder infection in an anuric or severely oliguric patient, it is extremely difficult to clear and often requires intervention, including surgery. Lastly, patients on both hemodialysis and peritoneal dialysis have an increased incidence of UTIs, and doubtless some are secondary to infections elsewhere [26].

Immunosuppression

Patients who are immunosuppressed, either by medications or by other comorbid conditions, must always be treated aggressively [27]. There are a number of drugs in which immunosuppression is the desired outcome, but a secondary effect is increased infections throughout the body, including the urinary tract. The prototype of these is corticosteroids. There are a number of ways that these drugs are delivered, namely orally, parenterally, nasally, cutaneously, and others. All cause immunosuppression in a dose dependent fashion by reducing the cell-mediated immune responses and local immune reaction. There is also an effect on the humoral immune system, although this is not as pronounced. Many drugs exist that are intended to abrogate the immune response (IR) caused by the condition being treated. Patients undergoing organ transplantation are the most obvious of the category, as they may be taking corticosteroids as well. Drugs such as the calcineurine inhibitors (cyclosporine and tacrolimus) are cell-mediated immunity specific [28,29]. Additionally, monoclonal antibodies are currently being used to treat transplant rejection, and have profound effects on the treatment of UTI. The immunosuppressant drugs, such as muromonab-CD3 and a host of others, fit into this category. The cell-cycle nonspecific drugs, such as azathioprine and mycophenolate mofetil, are also a concern, as they are not only used in treatment of organ transplantation, but also in other diseases.

Urolithiasis

Urolithiasis is certainly one of the medical conditions that confers the designation of "complicated" [30]. The most ominous complication of stones is obstruction. The association of an obstructing calculus along with febrile UTI is usually considered an emergency, because of the risk of sepsis. Intervention is mandatory in most cases, specifically by employing either a nephrostomy tube or a ureteral stent. Moreover, stones may prolong the treatment of UTIs if they are infected. The bacteria become ensconced in the interstices of the stone and, usually, by establishing their own biofilm environment [31], become difficult or even impossible to eradicate without removal of the calculus. Stones also cause injury to the urinary tract, and the damage can give bacteria a place to establish colonization. This is especially true if intervention has become necessary to effect calculus removal. Certain stones are a direct result of infections, specifically magnesium ammonium phosphate or calcium carbonate stones. Urea-splitting microorganisms, by altering their microenvironment, facilitate precipitation of these salts, promoting de novo stone formation and thus persistence of infection. If the bacteria come in contact with other types of stones and establish a nidus for infection, they may lay down new matrix upon the existing stone, creating an eclectic mix of calculus material.

Surgery of the urinary tract

Whenever surgery of the urinary tract becomes necessary, whether for obstruction, calculus, or other causes, the urinary tract becomes more susceptible to UTIs and persistence or recurrence thereof. Disruptions or irregularities of the urothelium may serve as an initiation point for UTIs or the creation of obstruction. The underlying abnormality may not have been entirely corrected, and originally may have been a risk factor for infection itself. Furthermore, from time to time sutures may persist in the urinary tract, even when the material is designed to dissolve. If sutures remain long enough, colonization may occur, and even stones have been observed. In the setting of a person presenting with a UTI, this history may be critical to the treatment and long-term management.

Functional and anatomical abnormalities of the urinary tract

There are a number of functional and anatomical abnormalities of the urinary tract that confer complicated status upon UTIs. Most of these are congenital and present early in life with imperfections or voiding dysfunction [32]. Vesico-ureteral reflux, ureteropelvic junction obstruction, urethral valves (anterior or posterior), and congenital megaureter are some of the most common of these abnormalities. All have been associated with an increased incidence of UTIs, as well as a need for prolonged antibiotic therapy or intervention. Correction of these abnormalities may reduce the risk of UTIs, but their occurrences in the setting of an infection implies a complicated label [33]. Other structural abnormalities include polycystic kidney disease, renal artery stenosis, renal vein varices or thrombosis, calyceal diverticula, medullary sponge kidney, and others. Whereas some of these may be corrected or near-corrected with surgery and medications, the risk for a complicated UTI remains greater in these cases than among the general population, and should be managed accordingly.

Pregnancy

Pregnancy always confers complicated status on any UTI [34,35]. The risk to the fetus alone would serve as an adequate descriptor, but it is even more complicated because of the pregnant woman's anatomic and endocrinologic milieu. The gravid uterus, depending of course on the trimester, will cause an anatomic alteration that involves a relative obstructive uropathy. It is unusual that drainage is needed, but this must always be a consideration. After clearance of the UTI, some decision regarding prophylactic antibiotics should be made. The hormone status also has a significant bearing on the infection management. A reduction in smooth muscle contractility, not only of the uterus, but also of the ureter and bladder, may confer a degree of obstructive uropathy. It has been shown that progesterone levels correlate closely with reduced ureteral motility and may both predispose to UTIs and prolong their treatment. The voiding dysfunction that almost invariably accompanies a pregnancy also negatively impacts the resistance to and treatment of UTIs. Most pregnant patients have frequency and urgency, along with stress incontinence, all leading to voiding dysfunction. For those circumstances where there is an increase in bladder pressure, this may lead to a reduction in the local defense mechanisms against UTI. Venous congestion may further contribute to the increased susceptibility. It has been shown that these conditions disrupt the tight junctions in the bladder epithelium, and that the uromucoid (a protective layer of mucus, Tamm-Horsfall protein, and other substances) is damaged by the high pressures and fails to protect.

Voiding dysfunction

Patients with voiding dysfunction, including those with neurogenic bladders, comprise a significant proportion of complicated UTIs [36–38]. Two characteristics of this problem are the prime reasons to be included in the group referred to as "complicated." The first of these is the frequent presence of residual urine. Conditions such as low spinal cord injury, myogenic atony, spina bifida, sacral agenesis, and a host of others may allow for incomplete emptying and thus an enhanced milieu for bacterial growth. This can also be a result of bladder outlet obstruction, either anatomic or physiologic. These conditions add the complication of high pressure voiding, which is the second characteristic. The high pressure contributes on several levels. The first is a reduction in blood supply, impairing IR and host response. Second, the high pressures disrupt the uromucoid layer and may separate the urothelial cells, all causing a facilitation of bacterial binding and ultimately colonization. Last, over time, bladder damage, with cellules and diverticula may emerge, as does secondary vesicoureteral reflux. These lead to incomplete emptying, which greatly contributes to the sequestration of bacteria, establishment of individual microbial ecosystems, and reduced clearance by drugs, as well as renal insufficiency.

Environment

The place where a particular UTI is acquired must be factored into the equation. Infections that are generated in the community at large tend to be uncomplicated [39,40]. The organisms that come from this vast pool are the most common because of their particular proclivity and survival advantages. Just because of the numbers alone the most common organisms will have an advantage. The more unusual or resistant bacteria have less of a survival advantage in the community at large, and thus are not as prevalent. Hospital acquired or nosocomial infections all must be considered complicated because of a host of factors [5,6,8,41]. The susceptible population is very large, and even their different susceptibilities tend to be greater and of more importance. Indwelling catheters and other breaks in the body's integument provide for initiation points of the infection. The enormous amount of antibiotics present in this environment not only selects bacteria that are resistant, but also exerts selective pressure on the environment as a whole, fostering emergence of greater and greater resistance. Hospitalized patients contracting UTIs are particularly worrisome, in that the mortality rate for this particular infection may be upwards of 30% [10].

Another location for complicated UTIs to break out is in nursing homes [42]. In this environment, not only are there a large number of highly susceptible patients in very close propinquity, but also many have a compromised genitourinary tract because of indwelling catheters, skin breakdown, or loss of urinary or bowel control with the attendant prolonged exposure. Another problem tends to be cross contamination from patient to patient transmitted by the health care providers themselves. Whereas increased attention focused on hand washing may reduce this to a degree, the number of chances for exposure are often overwhelming. As the population ages and this type of long-term care becomes increasingly prevalent and popular, these infections will certainly be perpetuated.

Occasionally patients who travel to certain parts of the globe may be exposed to an increased variety of infective agents. With the exceptions of sexually transmitted diseases and some very regional infections, such as schistosomiasis, these tend to be very unusual. Unusual pulmonary and dermatologic infections are much more commonly contracted in countries other than the United States. The involvement of the urinary tract is secondary to spread in a miliary fashion from the point of entry. In any case, the degree to which this type of infection contributes to the overall numbers is very small, although significant.

Pathogenic factors: organism-related factors contributing to complicated UTI

The organisms that are typically found in complicated UTIs are varied. The initial infection typically is caused by *Escherichia coli*. This organism is the most common facultative aerobic organism in the gastrointestinal tract, as it sits in proximity to the genitourinary tract. In addition, *E. coli* has a number of survival advantages to establishing a colony, and ultimately an infection, over other Gram-negative species. Many subtypes are imbued with surface structures that bind to specific locations on the urothelial cell surface. Perhaps the most important of these are fimbria, most notably type I fimbriae, which are inhibited by mannose and avidly bind to latex catheters and urothelial cells [12]. In addition, there are P-fimbriae, which bind to a urothelial cell surface receptor referred to as the P-blood group antigen present in the majority of the world population and located on the urothelial cells as well [12]. Because *E. coli* is the most common organism in the intestine, other than anaerobes, it stands to reason that it would be the most common in all types of UTIs, especially given its survival advantages. Those with the P-blood group antigen are able to ascend the urinary tract easily, even in the anatomically normal system.

A host of other Gram-negative species may also be found in the complicated UTI group. Many of these are nosocomially acquired, and as such will reflect the local hospital environment. These will be highly specific to the particular hospital or nursing home where the host is exposed. Because complete eradication is often a problem, and because the local microenvironment may undergo change based upon numerous factors, the individual patients may have more than one bacteria that is causing the UTI. These still are in the minority with one notable exception, namely the infection in the setting of an indwelling catheter that has contact with the outside (urethral or suprapubic catheter). Over time, multiple species may colonize the catheter, and thus the urine. Not all of these species are capable of causing a true infection, but they may complicate the circumstances in other ways.

One of these is the sharing of genetic material, both chromosomal or naked DNA, often in defined entities referred to as "plasmids." These are readily spread throughout a bacterial population by conjugation and other means, resulting in multiple antibiotic resistant infections [9]. As certain plasmids exert a survival advantage in the setting of antimicrobial drug treatment, the population may grow rather quickly. The main reasons that these highly resistant organisms don't proliferate outside the hospital environment are the lack of selective antibiotic pressure in the community, the high degree of dilution (given the much greater population), and the fact that maintenance of the specific resistance itself requires extra metabolic energy in a given bacterium. Thus, in the absence of specific antibiotics, the organism is actually at a survival disadvantage.

Another property of bacteria that causes certain species to have a great survival advantage is matrix or glycocalyx synthesis (also referred to as biofilm) [11,43,44]. Certain bacteria, the prototypic one being *Pseudomonas aeruginosa*, are able to synthesize a substance into their microenvironment, which forms a protective shell around themselves. This serves three major functions, all promoting survival. The first is protection from the body's immune response: the leukocytes cannot penetrate the covering and are rendered ineffectual. The second is exclusion of antibiotics that, if capable of penetrating this layer, may not be capable of concentrating there. An exception to this is the 5-fluoroquinolone ciprofloxacin [45]. The third property is that the bacteria have a much greater control over their microenvironment, concentrating nutrients, excluding toxic substances, preventing dilution of products needed for metabolism, all serving to allow the bacterium to stabilize and improve its metabolic rate. The advantage of this is to let it reduce its susceptibility to antibiotics or the IR in a state of relative hibernation, emerging when the external environment is more conducive to growth and division. The organisms capable of this synthesis are the same ones that tend to harbor antibiotic resistances as well.

Other than *Staphylococcus saprophyticus*, infections caused by Gram-positive species are more commonly seen in complicated UTI groups [8,13,33]. The occasional simple UTI will be caused by group D streptococci (enterococci), but not as commonly as the former. The reasons are that most of these species lack the external appendages to bind avidly to the urothelial cell surface, and thus have a lower probability of establishing a colony to initiate the infectious process. Second, they are not as ubiquitous in the area in and near the urethral opening. Similarly, they are not seen in the colon or mucosal surfaces either. Third, they often lack specific virulence factors for the urinary tract, to allow them to establish a colony and invade. One of the reasons that the Gram-positive organisms are grouped under the complicated UTI definition is that they may be spread via the hematogenous route, and they tend to be a result of a significant insult to the body's defense mechanisms. An example of this is *Staphylococcus aureus* infection, which often can come from an infected site elsewhere in the body, causing bacteremia and therefore seeding of the kidney [46]. This may also occur in the circumstance of an intravenous drug abuser or someone who has an infected indwelling line. These infections may progress to some of the significant sequelae of complicated UTIs, specifically lobar nephronia (renal carbuncle) or perinephric abscess, requiring long-term antibiotics or intervention, either endoscopic or surgical.

Another group of pathogens that are included in the complicated group are the fungi. The most common of this group, by far, is the genus *Candida*, with the species *albicans*, *tropicalis*, and *kruzei* predominating. These yeast forms are frequently found in the urinary tract as a colonizing agent, rather than an infecting organism [47]. It may, however, denote a polymicrobial urinary environment, and in the setting of an intubated urinary tract, may be of greater significance. In any case, *Candida* accounts for less than 5% of complicated UTIs. The other fungi comprise a very tiny percentage, with isolated case reports of prostatitis, pyelonephritis, and other infections caused by fungi other than *Candida*.

Evaluation of the patient with complicated UTI

Patients fitting the group of high risk for complicated UTI need an expeditious evaluation, specifically designed to limit the short and long-term morbidity and mortality. The first step in the priority of these patients is an accurate history and physical. This will help stratify the risks for the various confounding variables seen in this population. Secondly, a urine culture is mandatory, as opposed to uncomplicated UTIs, where empiric therapy is always instituted and frequently completed by the time a urine culture would be finalized. An assessment of the patient's general medical status, specifically hematologic profiles and complete serum chemistries, are usually required for management. Lastly, some imaging study should be mandatory, to discern whether other complicating issues coexist. This is especially true in patients who are known to have congenital malformations of the kidney and the immunocompromised or elderly. There was a time when ultrasound was probably the most desirous examination, because of cost, access, lack of radiation exposure, absence of contrast complications, and availability [48]. Most recently, computerized axial tomographic scanning (CT) has supplanted most of these tests, because the improved technology and advanced imaging, which has cut the acquisition time drastically. The CT also affords improved detail and image resolution, and can diagnose essentially all pathology identified by the ultrasound. Other studies may be necessary, but if either the ultrasound or CT is negative for correctable pathology, then other imaging studies are not warranted [49].

There are a number of sequela from complicated UTIs that may have serious or fatal consequences [50]. The most worrisome is urosepsis. While this is certainly more likely in immunocompromised patients, all patients with complicated UTIs are at risk. This is far more common with Gram-negative organisms and may be fatal. The hypotensive effects of the bacterial cell wall (endotoxin), coupled with a wide array of externally synthesized enzymes and other biologically active products, results in profound hemodynamic changes, multiple organ failure, and often death. Use of antibiotics in the environment for other problems further complicates the circumstances by limiting the available treatment options.

Another ominous side effect of complicated UTIs is renal failure. This may be acute or chronic and may be permanent or self-limited. Pre-existing renal insufficiency is a predisposing factor, as is obstruction. From there, abscesses may develop. One particular complication, emphysematous pyelonephritis, occurs in diabetics far more commonly than it does in patients with normal glucose control. This entity is characterized by the finding of air in the renal parenchyma, identified by CT, ultrasound, or abdominal radiographs. Intervention is always required and even if instituted in a timely fashion, there is a high mortality rate. Xanthogranulomatous pyelonephritis and malakoplakia are relatively uncommon complications, but almost always result in renal loss.

Treatment of the patient with complicated UTI

Several principles guide the treatment of complicated UTIs. The first of these is to minimize the effects of obstruction or other obfuscating anatomic abnormality. Relief of obstruction is the primary way this is accomplished, but others are employed as needed. Second, aggressive use of antibiotics is mandatory. This means appropriate use of broad-spectrum drugs in appropriate dosages, adjusted for renal or hepatic insufficiency [51,52]. It is always necessary to not only cover Gram-positive and Gram-negative bacteria, but also to choose the specific drugs based upon the antibiogram available in the hospital or area. It is probably appropriate to consider prophylactic coverage of yeast, at least empirically, especially with an indwelling catheter or in the diabetic patient. Once the cultures and sensitivities have returned, adjustments must be made to ensure coverage. The same effort should also be made to reduce the development of resistance [7,52,53]. This involves not overusing a particular agent or using it inappropriately. The older antibiotic agents (eg, penicillins and aminoglycosides) should remain as first-line options. This should preserve the activity of the newer agents (eg, newer generations of cephalosporins and so forth). The problem is that resistance will tend to increase to the older agents over time, rendering them less effective. A very effective modality is to use combination therapy, not only for the additive effects but also for potential synergy. This is especially true when antibiotics from different classes are used together, because they work on different sites in the bacterium. The clinician should employ agents that have an advantageous pharmacokinetic profile, and a better pharmacodynamic profile against the pathogens that are suspected.

There is a little doubt that complicated UTIs will continue to increase in prevalence, because of an increase in the subpopulations of patients who are at risk. The average age of citizens is increasing, as is the likelihood of contacting those diseases that are associated with aging. The treatments for these diseases, from diabetes to renal calculi continue to increase this pool. It is incumbent, then, on the medical community to not only diagnose this condition in an expeditious fashion, but also to treat aggressively and intelligently to not only shorten the disease course, but also to minimize antimicrobial resistance.

References

[1] Stamm WE, Hooton TM. Management of urinary tract infections in adults. N Engl J Med 1993;329: 1328–34.
[2] Kallenius G, Mollby R, Svenson SB, et al. Occurrence of P-fimbriated *Escherichia coli* in urinary tract infections. Lancet 1981;2:1369–72.

[3] Neal DE Jr, Dilworth P, Kaack MB, et al. Experimental prostatitis in nonhuman primates: II. Ascending acute prostatitis. Prostate 1990;17:233–9.

[4] Melekos MD, Naber KG. Complicated urinary tract infections. Int J Antimicrob Agents 2000;15:247–56.

[5] Bouza E, San Juan R, Munoz P, et al. European Study Group on Nosocomial Infections. A European Perspective on Nosocomial Urinary Tract Infections I. Report on the microbiology workload, etiology and antimicrobial susceptibility (ESGNI-003 study). Clin Microbiol Infect 2001;7:523–31.

[6] Sahm DF, Thornsberry C, Mayfield DC, et al. Multidrug-resistant urinary tract isolates of *Escherichia coli*: prevalence and patient demographics in the United States in 2000. Antimicrob Agents Chemother 2001;1402–6.

[7] Gupta K, Sahm DF, Mayfield D, et al. Antimicrobial resistance among uropathogens that cause community-acquired urinary tract infections in women: a nationwide analysis. Clin Infect Dis 2001;33: 88–94.

[8] Mathai D, Jones RN, Pfaller MA. Epidemiology and frequency of resistance among pathogens causing urinary tract infection in 1,510 hospitalized patients: a report from the SENTRY Antimicrobial Surveillance Program (North America). Diagn Microbiol Infect Dis 2001;40:129–36.

[9] Neal DE Jr, Moody EEM, Thomas VL, et al. In vivo transfer of an R-plasmid in a urinary tract infection model. J Urol 1989;141:1460–2.

[10] Nicolle LE. Urinary tract pathogens in complicated infection and in elderly individuals. J Infect Dis 2001;183(Suppl 1):S5–8, A.

[11] Nicolle LE. Catheter-related urinary tract infection. Drugs Aging 2005;22(8):627–39.

[12] Dowling KJ, Roberts JA, Kaack MB. P-fimbriated *E.Coli* urinary tract infection: a clinical correlation. South Med J 1987;80:1533–6.

[13] Foxman B. Epidemiology of urinary tract infections: incidence, morbidity, and economic costs. Am J Med 2002;113(Suppl 1a):5S–13S.

[14] Crawford ED, Wilson SS, McConnell JD, et al. Baseline factors as predictors of clinical progression of benign prostatic hyperplasia in men treated with placebo. J Urol 2006;175(4):1422–6. J Urol 1426–7.

[15] Fair WR, Couch J, Wehner N. Prostatic antibacterial factor. Identify and significance. Urology 1976; 7(2):169–77.

[16] Randolph JG. Congenital abnormalities of the urinary collecting system: their recognition and management. Pediatr Clin North Am 1965;12:381–409.

[17] Koff SA. Clues to neonatal genitourinary problems. Postgrad Med 1977;62(3):93–101.

[18] Singh-Grewal D, Macdessi J, Craig J. Circumcision for the prevention of urinary tract infection in boys: a systematic review of randomized trials and observational studies. Arch Dis Child 2005;90(8):853–8 [epub 2005 May 12].

[19] Ribera MC, Pascual R, Orozco D, et al. Incidence and risk factors associated with urinary tract infection in diabetic patients with and without asymptomatic bacteriuria. Eur J Clin Microbiol Infect Dis 2006;25(6):389–93.

[20] Hoepelman AI, Meiland R, Geerlings SE. Pathogenesis and management of bacterial urinary tract infections in adult patients with diabetes mellitus. Int J Antimicrob Agents 2003;22(Suppl 2):35–43.

[21] Stapleton A. Urinary tract infections in patients with diabetes. Am J Med 2002;(Suppl 1):80S–4S.

[22] Falagas ME, Alexiou VG, Giannopoulou KP, et al. Risk factors for mortality in patients with emphysematous pyelonephritis: a meta-analysis. J Urol 2007; 178(3):880–5 [epub 2007 Jul 16].

[23] Ooi ST, Frazee LA, Gardner WG. Management of asymptomatic bacteriuria in patients with diabetes mellitus. Ann Pharmacother 2004;38(3):490–3 [epub 2004 Jan 23].

[24] Moradi M, Abbasi M, Moradi A, et al. Effect of antibiotic therapy on asymptomatic bacteriruia in kidney transplant recipients. Urol J 2005;2(1):32–5.

[25] Pellé G, Vimont S, Levy PP. Acute pyelonephritis represents a risk factor impairing long-term kidney graft function. Am J Transplant 2007;7(4):899–907 [epub 2007 Feb7].

[26] Kamińska W, Patzer J, Dzierzanowska D. Urinary tract infections caused by endemic multi-resistant Enterobacter cloacae in a dialysis and transplantation unit. J Hosp Infect 2002;51(3):215–20.

[27] Tseng CC, Wu JJ, Liu HL, et al. Roles of host and bacterial virulence factors in the development of upper urinary tract infection caused by *Escherichia coli*. Am J Kidney Dis 2002;39(4):744–52.

[28] Maddux MS, Veremis SA, Bauma WD, et al. Effective prophylaxis of early post-transplant urinary tract infections (UTI) in the cyclosporine (CSA) era. Transplant Proc 1989;21(1 Pt 2):2108–9.

[29] Senger SS, Arslan H, Azap OK, et al. Urinary tract infections in renal transplant recipients. Transplant Proc 2007;39(4):1016–7.

[30] Conrad S, Busch R, Huland H. Complicated urinary tract infections. Eur Urol 1991;19(Suppl 1): 16–22.

[31] Ulett GC, Valle J, Beloin C, et al. Functional analysis of antigen 43 in uropathogenic *Escherichia coli* reveals a role in long-term persistence in the urinary tract. Infect Immun 2007;75(7):3233–44 [epub 2007 Apr 9].

[32] American Academy of Pediatrics. Practice parameter: the diagnosis, treatment, and evaluation of the initial urinary tract infection in febrile infants and young children. American Academy of Pediatrics. Committee on Quality Improvement. Subcommittee on Urinary Tract Infection. Pediatrics 1999; 103(4 pt 1):843–52.

[33] Hummers-Pradier E, Kochen MM. Urinary tract infections in adult general practice patients. Br J Gen Pract 2002;52:752–61.

[34] Bánhidy F, Acs N, Puhó EH, et al. Maternal urinary tract infection and related drug treatments during pregnancy and risk of congential abnormalities in the offspring. BJOG 2006;113(12):1465–71.

[35] McLaughlin SP, Carson CC. Urinary tract infections in women. Med Clin North Am 2004;88(2):417–29.

[36] Yeung CK, Sreedhar B, Leung YF, et al. Correlation between ultrasonographic bladder measurements and urodynamic findings in children with recurrent urinary tract infection. BJU Int 2007;99(3):651–5 [epub 2006 Nov 7].

[37] Shaikh N, Abedin S, Docimo SG. Can ultrasonography or uroflowmetry predict which children with voiding dysfunction will have recurrent urinary tract infections? J Urol 2005;174(4 Pt 2):1620–2 [discussion 1622].

[38] Okorocha I, Cummings G, Gould I. Female urodynamics and lower urinary tract infection. BJU Int 2002;89(9):863–7.

[39] Talan DA, Stamm WE, Hooton TM, et al. Comparison of ciprofloxacin (7 days) and trimethoprimsulfamethoxazole (14 days) for acute uncomplicated pyelonephritis in women: a randomized trial. JAMA 2000;283:1583–90.

[40] Warren JW, Abrutyn E, Hebel JR, et al. Guidelines for antimicrobial treatment of uncomplicated acute bacterial cystitis and acute pyelonephritis in women. Infectious Diseases Society of America (IDSA). Clin Infect Dis 1999;29:745–58.

[41] Gaynes R, Edwards JR. National Nosocomial Infections Surveillance System. Overview of nosocomial infections caused by gram-negative bacilli. Clin Infect Dis 2005;41:848–54.

[42] Regal RE, Pham CQ, Bostwick TR. Urinary tract infections in extended care facilities: preventive management strategies. Consult Pharm 2006;21(5):400–9.

[43] Soto SM, Smithson A, Horcajada JP, et al. Implication of biofilm formation in the persistence of urinary tract infection caused by uropathogenic Escherichia coli. Clin Microbiol Infect 2006;12(10):1034–6.

[44] Goto T, Nakame Y, Nishida M, et al. Bacterial biofilms and catheters in experimental urinary tract infection. Int J Antimicrob Agents 1999;11(3–4): 227–31.

[45] Rodríguez-Martínez JM, Ballesta S, Pascual A. Activity and penetration of fosfomycin, ciprofloxacin, amoxicillin/clauvulanic acid and co-trimoxazole in Escherichia coli and Pseudomonas aeruginosa biofilms. Int J Antimicrob Agents 2007;30(4):366–8.

[46] Ekkelenkamp MB, Verhoef J, Bonten MJ. Quantifying the relationship between Staphylococcus aureus bacteremia and S. aureus bacteriuria: a retrospective analysis in a tertiary care hospital. Clin Infect Dis 2007;44(11):1457–9 [epub 2007 Apr 18].

[47] Sobel JD, Kauffman CA, McKinsey D, et al. Candiduria: a randomized double-blind study of treatment with fluconazole and placebo. The National Institute of Allergy and Infectious Diseases (NIAID) Mycoses Study Group. Clin Infect Dis 2000;30:19–24.

[48] Neal DE Jr, Steele R, et al. Ultrasonography in the differentiation of complicated and uncomplicated acute pyelonephritis. Am J Kidney Dis 1990;16(5): 478–80.

[49] Neal DE Jr, Steele R. The role of CT scanning in evaluation of common renal lesions. Infections in Urology 1992;5(2):37–45.

[50] Neal DE Jr. Host defense mechanisms in urinary tract infections. Infections in Urol. Urol Clin North Am 1999;26(4):677–86.

[51] Carson C, Naber KG. Role of fluoroquinolones in the treatment of serious bacterial urinary tract infections. Drugs 2004;64:1359–73.

[52] Nicolle LE. A practical guide to antimicrobial management of complicated urinary tract infection. Drugs Aging 2001;18:243–54.

[53] Zhanel GG, Hisanaga TL, Laing NM, et al. Antibiotic resistance in outpatient urinary isolates. final results from the North American Urinary Tract Infection Collaborative Alliance (NAUTICA). Int J Antimicrob Agents 2005;26:380–8.

ELSEVIER
SAUNDERS

Urol Clin N Am 35 (2008) 23–32

UROLOGIC
CLINICS
of North America

Bacterial Prostatitis

Brian M. Benway, MD[a], Timothy D. Moon, MBChB, FRCSC[a,b],*

[a]*Division of Urology, Department of Surgery, University of Wisconsin Hospital-Medical School,
600 Highland Avenue, Room G5/341 CSC, Madison, WI 53792, USA*
[b]*Veterans Affairs Medical Center, Clinical Science Center, 600 Highland Avenue, Madison, WI 53792-3236, USA*

Prostatitis in all its manifestations places a significant strain on patients and urologists. It is perhaps the most common urologic complaint in men younger than 50 years of age [1] and affects 11% to 16% of American men over the course of their lifetimes [2,3]. Prostatitis syndromes have a significant psychologic impact upon patients who suffer from them and place an enormous financial strain upon the health care system [4,5]. Despite many advances in our understanding of the pathogenesis and treatment of prostatitis, current management strategies are unable to provide a significant portion of relief from the symptoms of prostatitis.

In the 1999 NIH consensus statement on prostatitis, prostatitis and prostatitis-like symptoms were classified into four broad categories (Table 1) [6]. Type I prostatitis refers to acute bacterial prostatitis. Type II prostatitis encompasses chronic bacterial prostatitis. Type III is the most common manifestation of the syndrome, affecting 90% of patients diagnosed with prostatitis, and is characterized by chronic pelvic pain in the absence of detectable infection. Type IV prostatitis refers to asymptomatic inflammation, found incidentally at the time of surgery, biopsy, or autopsy.

Acute bacterial prostatitis and chronic bacterial prostatitis represent only a small proportion of prostatitis cases. Type I prostatitis is the most

rare—it is diagnosed in less than 0.02% of all patients seen for prostatitis [7]—, but the potential morbidity and mortality of acute prostatitis constitute a true urologic emergency.

Type II prostatitis affects 5% to 10% of patients who have chronic prostatitis. Many patients are diagnosed with recurrent urinary tract infections with the same organism and often have detectable pathogens in prostatic secretions during asymptomatic periods [6].

In this article, we focus on bacterial prostatitis (types I and II), with an emphasis on new understandings of pathogenesis, diagnosis, and treatment strategies for these often challenging patients.

Acute bacterial prostatitis

Presentation and diagnosis

Acute bacterial prostatitis constitutes a urologic emergency. Upon presentation, patients are often acutely ill and in distress. These patients have obvious signs and symptoms of a urinary tract infection, including dysuria and urinary frequency [6]. They often present with intense suprapubic pain, urinary obstruction, fever, malaise, arthralgia, and myalgia [6–8].

Although a gentle rectal examination can be performed in patients who have suspected acute bacterial prostatitis, prostatic massage is inadvisable because it could precipitate bacteremia or frank sepsis [8]. Expressed prostatic secretion (EPS) or voided bladder 3 urine (VB3) are not necessary because the diagnosis can be made largely on symptomatic presentation. Although prostate-specific antigen (PSA) levels are not

* Corresponding author. Department of Surgery, Division of Urology, University of Wisconsin Hospital-Medical School, 600 Highland Avenue, Room G5/341 CSC, Madison, WI 53792.

E-mail address: moon@surgery.wisc.edu (T.D. Moon).

0094-0143/08/$ - see front matter. Published by Elsevier Inc.
doi:10.1016/j.ucl.2007.09.008

urologic.theclinics.com

Table 1
National Institutes of Health classification of prostatitis
syndromes

Category I	Acute bacterial prostatitis
Category II	Chronic bacterial prostatitis
Category III: chronic pelvic pain syndrome (CPPS)	Chronic pelvic pain without the presence of bacteria localized to the prostate
Category III a: inflammatory CPPS	Presence of significant numbers of white blood cells in expressed prostatic secretion
Category IIIb	Insignificant numbers of white blood cells in expressed prostatic secretion
Category IV: Asymptomatic inflammatory prostatitis	White blood cells in expressed prostatic secretion or histologic inflammation in prostatic tissue in asymptomatic individuals

a mainstay of diagnosis, they are generally moderately to markedly elevated in the setting of acute bacterial prostatitis [9–11].

For patients in whom a prostatic abscess is suspected, CT scan or careful transrectal ultrasound after initiation of antimicrobial therapy can aid in the diagnosis or exclusion of a prostatic abscess without increasing the risk for urosepsis [12,13].

Management

Appropriate management of acute bacterial prostatitis includes rapid initiation of broad-spectrum parenteral antibiotics and symptomatic support (Fig. 1) [14]. Typical treatment is with a penicillin or penicillin derivative, with the addition of an aminoglycoside. After successful initial therapy, patients can be transitioned to oral antibiotics (eg, fluoroquinolines), with a suggested minimum duration of three to four weeks. The long-term response is unclear. Figures of 90% have been reported [15], although a prospective study found a bacterial persistence rate at 3 months of 33% [14]. Therefore, prolonged therapy of fluoroquinolines for 6 weeks and reevaluation after that has been recommended [14].

Because patients can have significant obstruction from an acutely inflamed prostate, bladder scanning for postvoid residual urine is recommended. If the residual urine is less than 100 mL, the patient should be initiated on alpha blocker therapy; if the residual is large, consideration

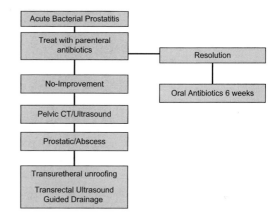

Fig. 1. Treatment algorithm for acute bacterial prostatitis.

should be given to placement of a small urethral catheter if short-term drainage is required or a suprapubic catheter if longer-term drainage is required [7]. Stool softeners are also recommended [8].

Special considerations for the immunocompromised patient

Patients who are immunocompromised, especially patients who have HIV/AIDS, seem to be more susceptible to the development of acute bacterial prostatitis and to the occurrence of a potentially life-threatening prostatic abscess [16]. Although the incidence of acute prostatitis in patients who have well controlled HIV is roughly equivalent to that of the general noncompromised population, the incidence rate rises to roughly 14% in those who have developed AIDS [16]. However, these data are quite old. Original studies updating these data during the last 8 years are lacking, and all current references refer back to the 1989 report [16]. It is these authors' impression that current rates are lower. If a prostatic abscess is discovered, initiation of broad-spectrum antibiotics and prompt surgical drainage is crucial.

Prostatic abscess

Prostatic abscesses are uncommon but potentially serious manifestations of acute infection of the prostate and demand prompt treatment. Patients who have a prostatic abscess are commonly immunocompromised or diabetic and typically present in a similar fashion to patients who have acute bacterial prostatitis without abscess, although unusual presentations do occur, as illustrated by a patient who presented with priapism [16,17]. Although CT and MRI are effective modalities for the diagnosis of prostatic abscess, transrectal ultrasound has been increasingly recommended due to its high sensitivity, greater cost-effectiveness, and ability to provide diagnosis and directed treatment in a single procedure, with CT being used primarily in cases where the transrectal ultrasound is nondiagnostic or suggestive of more extensive involvement [12,18,19].

Recommended treatment consists of broad-spectrum antibiotic coverage and, in most cases, drainage of the abscess. Although transurethral unroofing and perineal drainage were once the mainstays of surgical drainage, transrectal ultrasound-guided aspiration of prostatic abscesses has been increasingly used as an effective means of drainage that may avoid the potential morbidity associated with transurethral drainage [18,19]. Some authors also support urinary diversion with a suprapubic catheter [20,21].

Escherichia coli and *Staphylococcus* species are the most commonly isolated pathogens in prostatic abscess, although other pathogens, such as *Mycobacterium tuberculosis*, Actinomyces, Citrobacter, *Bacteroides fragilis*, *Aeromonas aerophyla*, and *Klebsiella pneumonia* have been reported [19–24]. *Burkholderia pseudomallei* overwhelmingly predominates in the Thai population [23].

Postbiopsy prostatitis

One of the most serious complications of transrectal biopsy of the prostate is the development of postbiopsy prostatitis and septicemia. Although these complications are rare, the severity of symptoms often necessitates an inpatient admission for administration of broad-spectrum intravenous antibiotics.

Bacteremia is common after prostate biopsy. A recent report found bacteremia in 44% patients undergoing transrectal biopsy without preprocedural antibiotics [25]. With proper antibiotic prophylaxis, generally with a single dose of a fluoroquinoline, infectious complications are likely to develop in only 1% to 2% of patients undergoing transrectal biopsy [26]. Studies also demonstrated no difference in efficacy between single-dose antibiotics given 2 hours before or at the time of biopsy [26]. Factors that increase the likelihood of infectious complications are the presence of an indwelling catheter and bactiuria at the time of biopsy [26].

It is generally agreed that antibiotic prophylaxis before biopsy is warranted, although the timing may not be critical. In addition, one study found that postbiopsy administration, although not recommended, is effective in preventing infectious complications [25]. The role of prebiopsy enema is a matter of debate. Although the data are mixed, the preponderance of evidence suggests that a prebiopsy enema is not beneficial when patients are given preprocedural antibiotics [26,27].

In the small proportion of patients who have no contraindication to biopsy in whom infectious complications develop despite antibiotic prophylaxis, resistant bacterial strains are a likely culprit. Of growing importance are multidrug resistant strains of *E coli* that escape traditional quinolone therapy. Known risk factors for colonization with resistant strains of *E coli* are age, travel to developing countries, and, most importantly, prior exposure to quinolones [28]. A case study found resistant strains of *Klebsiella* and *Pseudomonas* in a patient who developed multisystem organ failure after prostate biopsy [29].

Chronic bacterial prostatitis

Presentation

Classically, chronic bacterial prostatitis presents as recurrent urinary tract infection, usually with the same organism. Patients are not ill appearing but may complain of irritative voiding symptoms and testicular, lower back, or perineal discomfort [8]. On examination, the prostate may be palpably normal but may also have appreciable bogginess or tenderness [8]. Of patients who have chronic prostatitis, only 5% to 10% have evidence of infection [7].

Between episodes of urinary tract infection, bacterial infection in chronic bacterial prostatitis can be localized to the prostate, indicating ongoing prostatic infection [30]. Localization, historically, has involved the collection of multiple urine samples and expressed prostatic secretions to pinpoint the source of bacteria in patients who have prostatitis. Most urologists rely upon simplified diagnostic measures to localize bacteria in the urinary tract [31,32].

The four-glass versus the two-glass test

Classically, the diagnosis of prostatitis has hinged upon the gold-standard four-glass test, initially described by Mears and Stamey [31]. The four-glass test involves collection of distinct specimens, each designed to localize inflammation and infection to a distinct portion of the urinary tract. The VB1 specimen, or the initial 10 mL voided volume, localizes the urethra and can detect urethral colonization. The VB2 specimen corresponds to the standard midstream specimen and localizes to the bladder. The final two specimens are designed to directly examine the prostatic contents. For the third specimen, prostatic massage is performed, and the EPS are collected. Finally, the VB3, which is the first 10 mL of voided volume after prostatic massage, is collected; this specimen likely includes EPS that remains in the urethra after prostatic massage.

Few urologists perform the four-glass test, instead relying upon a two-glass test comprised of a midstream specimen and a postmassage specimen corresponding to the VB2 and VB3 portions of the four-glass test, respectively. A survey of urologists [32] found that few urologists (<20%) perform the standard four-glass test, with few attempting to obtain EPS samples. Moreover, a majority of urologists treat all forms of prostatitis empirically with antibiotics without performing a complete diagnostic test [32]. This has led to increased scrutiny of the "standard" diagnostic methods for prostatitis and to closer inspection of the necessity and practicality of performing the four-glass test.

A direct comparison of the sensitivity of the standard four-glass test compared with the two-glass test found the two-glass test to be 96% to 98% as accurate as the four-glass test, with the VB3 specimen failing to predict positive EPS specimens in a small number of patients [33]. Therefore, it could be argued based upon this evidence that the two-glass test is emerging as the appropriate new standard of evaluation.

One study has identified an alternate "two-glass" evaluation using VB1 samples combined with semen culture [34]. The authors note that semen culture is more sensitive than EPS in identifying gram-negative and gram-positive organisms, and semen sample collection forgoes potentially unnecessary discomfort associated with collection of VB3 or EPS through prostatic massage. In this study, gram-positive localization was highly inconsistent. An overall comparison of techniques is illustrated in Table 2.

Pathogenesis of chronic bacterial prostatitis

Classically, chronic bacterial prostatitis has been believed to be almost exclusively associated with infections due to uropathogenic gram-negative bacteria, most commonly *E coli*, but also Klebsiella SP, Proteus SPP, Pseudomonas, Aeruginosa, and more recently Enterococcus [30]. A growing amount of literature has focused on the role of other organisms, namely gram-positive bacteria and possibly anaerobes in the pathogenesis of prostatitis [35]. The FDA has accepted gram-positive organisms localized to the prostate as pathogens for the purpose of defining antimicrobial efficacy [36]. *E coli* is believed to be the most common pathogen in bacterial prostatitis, with enterococcus species ranking not far behind [37].

Recent studies have suggested that gram-positive bacteria may have a critical role in bacterial prostatitis, with some suggesting that the prevalence is higher than that of gram-negative species, the most common of which are *Enterococcus faecalis* and coagulase-negative staphylococcus species, such as *Staphylococcus aureus*, *S epidermidis*, and *S saprophyticus* [36,38,39]. *Corynebacterium* species have also been implicated, as has *S agalactiae* [30,40].

One study found that localization of gram-positive pathogens is largely inconsisten, and that the same gram-positive pathogen is rarely localized on repeated evaluation of untreated patients. Furthermore, patients who receive directed antimicrobial therapy for gram-positive cultures infrequently experience symptomatic relief. These data suggest that gram-positive species may represent specimen contamination or transient colonization of the urethra with what may represent normal flora [30].

One recent publication from the chronic prostatitis collaborative research network involved 463 patients and 121 age-matched control subjects for bacteria localized to the prostate [41]. Overall, 70% of patients and 76% of control subjects grew some organism. The growth of uropathogens was 8% for patients and 8.3% for control subjects.

Other organisms, such as *Ureaplasma urealyticum*, *Mycoplasma genitalium*, *Trichomonas vaginalis*, and *Chlamydia trachomatis*, have been isolated in the genitourinary tract of patients who suffer from bacterial prostatitis and may represent an underappreciated host of pathogens in the diagnosis of bacterial prostatitis [42–45]. Recent evidence suggests that prostatitis resulting from *C trachomatis* infections is sharply declining due to safer-sex practices in the HIV era or to better diagnosis and treatment of chlamydial infections by primary care providers before referral to an urologist [46].

Table 2
Evaluation of patients who have chronic bacterial prostatitis

	Mears-Stamey	Chronic Prostatitis Collaborative Research Network Study Group (CPCRN)	Budia [34]
Voided bladder 1 (initial stream urine culture)	X	–	X
Voided bladder 2 (mid-stream urine culture)	X	X	
Expressed prostatic secretion (culture)	X	–	
Voided bladder 3 post-prostatic massage culture (10 mL)	X	X	
Semen culture	–	–	X
Benefits of technique	Gold standard	46% concordance with Mears-Stamey	Possibly 15% more accurate than CPCRN technique
	Expensive	Cheaper	Cheaper

Evidence has suggested that for patients in whom *E coli*, *P mirabilis*, *K pneumoniae*, *Enterococcus* species, and *S agalactiae* are localized, there is often a concomitant elevation of white blood cells in EPS or VB3 specimens, whereas in patients who have localized infections of *C trachomatis*, *U urealyticum*, and *T vaginalis*, the white blood cell count in EPS and VB3 is normal [40].

Biofilms and virulence factors

Of the pathogens linked to bacterial prostatitis, perhaps *E coli* is the best studied. Growing evidence suggests that *E coli* strains that are common to prostatitis have enhanced pathogenicity over *E coli* strains that cause simple urinary tract infections or pyelonephritis [47–49].

Biofilm formation is considered an important feature that contributes to the relative impenetrability of *E coli* within the prostate. Biofilms are defined as colonies of bacteria that are densely adherent to one another and that are enveloped in a gelatinous matrix that serves as a barrier to immune and antibacterial response [47,48,50,51]. Two recent studies have demonstrated that *E coli* strains associated with bacterial prostatitis have a greater degree of biofilm formation than strains associated with cystitis and pyelonephritis, which may explain the fastidious nature of *E coli* within the prostate [47,48].

Other studies have found that, overall, *E coli* strains responsible for bacterial prostatitis exhibit more virulence factors than other uropathogenic *E coli*, including hemolysin and cytotoxic necrotizing factor [47,49]. These markers for increased virulence of pathogenic *E coli* help to explain why prostatitis remains difficult to treat despite the high vascularity of the prostate.

Special considerations for the immunocompromised patient

The immunocompromised patient represents a particular diagnostic and therapeutic challenge. Although patients who have HIV and AIDS are susceptible to the common pathogens found in noncompromised patients, species such as *Serratia marcescens*, *Salmonella typhi*, *M tuberculosis*, and *M avium* have been localized. In addition, nonbacterial pathogens (eg, HIV and cytomegalovirus) and fungi, including *Candida albicans*, *Apergillus fumigatus*, *Cryptococcus neoformans*, and *Histoplasma capsulatum*, have been found [52–55].

Current recommendations for the evaluation and treatment of chronic bacterial prostatitis in HIV-positive patients who have no prostatic abscess is 4 to 6 weeks, followed by low-dose suppressive antibiotics, the length of which has not been agreed upon [12,56].

Treatment of chronic bacterial prostatitis

Antibiotics

Antimicrobial therapy is a mainstay of treatment for chronic bacterial prostatitis, although not all antibiotics are equal (Fig. 2). Delivery of antimicrobials to the prostate is a passive process, whereby antibiotics diffuse into and concentrate in the prostate [57]. Factors affecting prostatic penetrance include molecular shape and size, drug–protein binding, lipid solubility, pH gradients, and ionization [7,58].

Fluoroquinolones have been generally shown to have the best penetrance into the prostate and seminal fluid [7,58]. In cases of chronic bacterial prostatitis that present with concurrently elevated PSA levels (~20% of patients who have chronic bacterial prostatitis), quinolones have been shown to decrease PSA levels; moreover, decreases in PSA levels in these patients was a positive predictor of symptomatic resolution and antimicrobial success [10]. As such, most researchers recommend fluoroquinolones as first-line antimicrobials in the treatment of chronic bacterial prostatitis [7,58].

Ciprofloxacin and levofloxacin are the most widely used quinolones in the treatment of chronic bacterial prostatitis. Although ciprofloxacin has a relatively low seminal fluid concentration compared with other quinolones, the prostatic fluid concentrations are high, which affords it reasonable efficacy [7,58]. Levofloxacin has some advantage over ciprofloxacin in that it achieves a higher concentration in prostatic fluid but not in ejaculate, spermatozoa, or seminal fluid [7,58,59].

Although penicillin derivatives have a reported role in the treatment of acute bacterial prostatitis, one study found that no patients treated with amoxicillin/clavulanic acid had resolution of their prostatitis [7,60].

Other antibiotic groups, such as doxycycline and macrolides, are considered second-line drugs [61]. The recommended duration of antimicrobial therapy is a matter of debate, but evidence suggests that a minimum course of 4 weeks is necessary for treatment of chronic bacterial prostatitis, although only weak support was noted in cases of gram-positive infection [35]. Response rates for trials conducted over the past several decades report response rates ranging from 0% to 100% [61]. More recent fluoroquinoline studies demonstrate efficacy, in terms of bacterial eradication, of 51% to 100% [61].

Alpha blockers

Although obstructive symptoms are common in patients who have acute bacterial prostatitis,

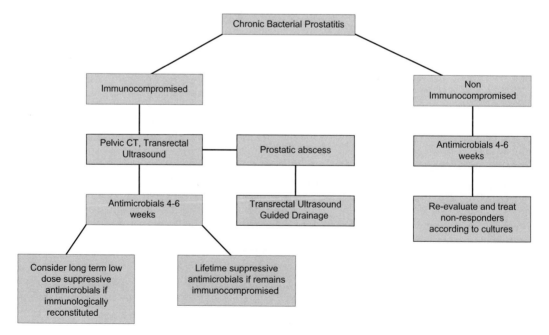

Fig. 2. Treatment algorithm for chronic bacterial prostatitis.

obstructive symptoms can be found in patients who have chronic bacterial prostatitis as well. Some authors support the notion that dysfunctional voiding or high resistance through the prostatic urethra may precipitate bacterial prostatitis by allowing for intraprostatic ductal reflux to deliver bacteria to the prostate [62,63]. Furthermore, obstructive symptoms may persist long after the bacterial infection has been cleared [62].

Alpha blockers have been investigated as an adjunct to antimicrobial therapy by Barbalias and colleagues [64]. Patients who had chronic bacterial prostatitis who received a combination of antibiotics and alpha blockers, compared with antibiotics alone, had a statistically significant increase in symptomatic relief and a significant decrease in relapse symptomatically and by objective culture data. The combination group experienced a quicker resolution of symptoms and a longer duration of symptomatic relief. The precise place for alpha blockers in category II and III prostatitis remains unclear. A recent study published by the Chronic Prostatitis Collaborative Research Network Study Group found no difference between fluoroquinoline, alpha blockers, or a combination [65], although the patients were heavily pretreated.

Prostatic massage

Prostatic massage was once an unqualified mainstay of treatment for chronic bacterial prostatitis, especially before the advent of effective antimicrobial therapy [60,66]. Prostatic massage is believed to be of aid in the treatment of prostatitis through a variety of proposed but unproven mechanisms. Rat models have demonstrated that in prostatitis, the infection is focused along the base of the glands [67]. Other studies have shown that ductal obstruction is closely linked to prostatitis [68,69] and that bacterial biofilms may inhibit antimicrobial penetrance [48,50,51]. Prostatic massage may help assist drainage by mechanically relieving ductal and acinar obstruction [60]. Massage may also improve antimicrobial efficacy by disrupting bacterial biofilms and by increasing prostatic blood flow and therefore delivery of antibiotic [60].

One study focusing on prostatic massage in conjunction with antimicrobial therapy found that over 80% of patients receiving combination therapy had at least a partial response, and 46% had a complete response. Response to combination therapy was positively predicted by positive pretreatment cultures, indicating a greater efficacy in type II versus type III patients. The study lacked a control group; therefore, the contribution made by prostatic massage cannot be qualified [60]. One controlled study found that combination therapy with prostatic massage and antibiotics offers no significant therapeutic benefit over directed antimicrobial therapy alone [70]. Overall opinions about prostatic massage are mixed [71].

Prostatitis and implications for other diseases of the prostate

Although studies to date have been correlative in nature, it seems evident that prostatitis is associated with other diseases of the prostate. An investigation of pathologic specimens of patients undergoing transurethral resection of the prostate for benign prostate hyperplasia demonstrated evidence of inflammation in nearly all specimens [70].

An investigation into the past medical histories of patients in Olmsted County, Minnesota, found that patients diagnosed with prostate cancer were more likely to have a prior diagnosis of prostatitis. Although the correlation with chronic prostatitis was weak, a stronger association was found between a history of acute prostatitis and prostate cancer diagnosis, with a mean interval of 12.2 years between the diagnosis of acute prostatitis and prostate cancer. The study may be confounded by the possibility that patients who have acute prostatitis may seek medical attention more readily, thus increasing the likelihood of prostate cancer detection in the absence of any true causative connection [72,73].

Summary

Bacterial prostatitis represents a small portion of the prostatitis spectrum. Acute bacterial prostatitis remains rare, although it is more common in the HIV/AIDS population where prostatic abscesses are more common. Abscesses have traditionally been drained transurethrally, although there seems to be a trend to transrectal ultrasound-guided drainage.

Chronic bacterial prostatitis also remains a small part of the prostatitis spectrum. Treatment remains primarily with antibiotics. The main dilemma remains classification as to whether

gram-positive bacteria are involved in the pathogenesis of chronic bacterial prostatitis.

References

[1] McNaughton Collins M, Stafford RS, O'Leary MP,
    et al. How common is prostatitis? A national survey
    of physician visits. J Urol 1998;159:1224–8.
[2] Roberts RO, Lieber MM, Rhodes T, et al. Preva-
    lence of a physician-assigned diagnosis of prostatitis:
    the Olmstead County study of urinary symptoms
    and health status among men. Urology 1998;1:
    578–84.
[3] McNaughton Collins M, Meigs JB, Barry MJ, et al.
    Prevalence and correlates of prostatitis in the health
    professionals follow-up study cohort. J Urol 2002;
    167:1363–6.
[4] McNaughton Collins M, Pontari MA, O'leary MP,
    et al. Quality of life is impaired in men with chronic
    prostatitis. J Gen Intern Med 2001;16:656–62.
[5] Calhoun EA, McNaughton Collins M, Pontari MA,
    et al. The economic impact of chronic prostatitis.
    Arch Intern Med 2004;164:1231–6.
[6] Krieger JN, Nyberg L, Nickel JC. NIH consensus
    definition and classification of prostatitis. JAMA
    1999;281(3):236–7.
[7] Wagenlehner FME, Weidner W, Sörgel F, et al. The
    role of antibiotics in chronic bacterial prostatitis. Int
    J Antimicrob Agents 2005;26:1–7.
[8] Roberts RO, Lieber MM, Bostwick DG, et al. A re-
    view of clinical and pathological prostatitis syn-
    dromes. Urology 1997;49(6):809–21.
[9] Hara N, Koike H, Ogino S, et al. Application of se-
    rum PSA to identify acute bacterial prostatitis in pa-
    tients with fever of unknown origin or symptoms of
    acute pyelonephritis. Prostate 2004;60:282–8.
[10] Schaeffer AJ, Wu S, Tennenberg AM, et al. Treat-
    ment of chronic bacterial prostatitis with levofloxa-
    cin and ciprofloxacin lowers serum prostate specific
    antigen. J Urol 2005;174:161–4.
[11] Neal DE Jr, Clejan S, Sarma D, et al. Prostate spe-
    cific antigen and prostatitis. I: effect of prostatitis
    on serum PSA in the human and nonhuman primate.
    Prostate 1992;20(2):105–11.
[12] Santillo VM, Lowe FC. The management of chronic
    prostatitis in men with HIV. Curr Urol Rep 2006;4:
    313–9.
[13] Horcajada JP, Vilana R, Moreno-Martínez A, et al.
    Transrectal prostatic ultrasonography in acute bac-
    terial prostatitis: findings and clinical implications.
    Scand J Infect Dis 2003;35:114–20.
[14] Kravchick S, Cryton S, Agulansky L, et al. Acute
    prostatitis in middle-aged men: a prospective study.
    BJU Int 2004;93:93–6.
[15] Schaeffer AJ. NIDDK-sponsored chronic prostati-
    tis collaborative research network (CPCRN) 5-
    year data and treatment guidelines for bacterial
    prostatitis. Int J Antimicrob Agents 2004;24S:
    S49–52.

[16] Leport C, Rousseau R, Perrone C, et al. Bacterial
    prostatitis in patients infected with the human im-
    munodeficiency virus. J Urol 1989;141(2):334–6.
[17] Shah J, Saleem M, Ellis BW. Prostate abscess pre-
    senting as priapism. Int J Clin Pract Suppl 2005;
    147:118–20.
[18] Göğüş Ç, Özden E, Karaboğa R, et al. The value of
    transrectal ultrasound guided needle aspiration in
    treatment of prostatic abscess. Eur J Radiol 2004;
    52:94–8.
[19] Chou Y, Tiu C, Liu J, et al. Prostatic abscess: trans-
    rectal color doppler ultrasonic diagnosis and
    minimally invasive therapeutic management. Ultra-
    sound Med Biol 2004;30(6):719–24.
[20] Ludwig M, Schroeder-Printzen S, Schiefer HS, et al.
    Diagnosis and therapeutic management of 18 patients
    with prostatic abscess. Urology 1999;53(2):340–5.
[21] Varkarakis J, Sebe P, Pinggera G, et al. Three-
    dimensional ultrasound guidance for percutaneous
    drainage of prostatic abscesses. Urology 2004;
    63(6):1017–20.
[22] Olivera P, Andrade JA, Port HC, et al. Diagnosis
    and treatment of prostatic abscess. Int Braz J Urol
    2003;29(1):30–4.
[23] Aphinives C, Pacheerat K, Chaiyakum J, et al. Pros-
    tatic abscesses: radiographic findings and treatment.
    J Med Assoc Thai 2004;87(7):810–5.
[24] Tai H. Emphysematous prostatic abscess: a case
    report and review of literature. J Infect 2007;54:
    e51–4.
[25] Lindert KA, Kabalin JN, Terris MK. Bacteremia
    and bacteriuria after transrectal ultrasound guided
    prostate biopsy. J Urol 2000;164:76–80.
[26] Lindstedt S, Lindstrom U, Ljunggren E, et al. Sin-
    gle-dose antibiotic prophylaxis in core prostate bi-
    opsy: impact of timing and identification of risk
    factors. Eur Urol 2006;50(4):832–7.
[27] Carey JM, Korman HJ. Transrectal ultrasound
    guided biopsy of the prostate: do enemas decrease
    clinically significant complications? J Urol 2001;
    166:82–5.
[28] Davidson AJ, Lawrentschuk N, Jennens ID, et al.
    Multi-resistant Escherichia coli speticaemia follow-
    ing transrectal ultrasound guided prostate biopsy:
    an emerging risk [abstract 65]. Br J Hosp Med
    (Lond) 2006;67(2):98–9.
[29] Gilad J, Borer A, Maimon N, et al. Failure of cipro-
    floxacin prophylaxis for ultrasound guided transrec-
    tal prostatic biopsy in the era of multiresistant
    enterobacteriaceae. J Urol 1999;161(1):222.
[30] Krieger JN, Ross SO, Limaye AP, et al. Inconsistent
    localization of gram-positive bacteria to prostate-
    specific specimens from patients with chronic prosta-
    titis. Urology 2005;66(4):721–5.
[31] Mears E, Stamey T. Bacteriologic localization pat-
    terns in bacterial prostatitis and urethritis. Invest
    Urol 1968;5:492–518.
[32] McNaughton Collins M, Fowler FJ, Elliott DB,
    et al. Diagnosing and treating chronic prostatitis:

do urologists use the four-glass test? Urology 2000; 55(3):403–7.

[33] Nickel JC, Shokses D, Wang Y, et al. How does the pre-massage and post-massage 2-glass test compare to the Meares-Stamey 4-glass test in mend with chronic prostatitis/chronic pelvic pain syndrome? J Urol 2006;176(1):119–24.

[34] Budia A, Palmero JL, Broseta E, et al. Value of semen culture in the diagnosis of chronic bacterial prostatitis: a simplified method. Scand J Urol Nephrol 2006;40:326–31.

[35] Nickel JC, Moon T. Chronic bacterial prostatitis: an evolving clinical enigma. Urology 2005;66:2–8.

[36] Bundrick W, Heron SP, Ray P, et al. Levofloxacin versus ciprofloxacin in the treatment of chronic bacterial prostatitis: a randomized double-blind multicenter study. Urology 2003;62:537–41.

[37] Cox CE, Childs SJ. Treatment of chronic bacterial prostatitis with temafloxacin. Am J Med 1991;91: 134S–9S.

[38] Nickel JC, Costerton JW. Coagulase-negative staphylococcus in chronic prostatitis. J Urol 1992;147: 398–400.

[39] Bergman B. On the relevance of gram-positive bacteria in prostatitis. Infection 1994;22(Suppl 1):S22.

[40] Skerk V, Krhen I, Schonwald S, et al. The role of unusual pathogens in prostatitis syndrome. Int J Antimicrob Agents 2004;24S:S53–6.

[41] Nickel JC, Alexander RB, Schaeffer AJ, et al. Leukocytes and bacteria in men with chronic bacterial prostatitis/chronic pelvic pain syndrome compared to asymptomatic controls. J Urol 2003;170:818–22.

[42] Shurbaji MS, Gupta PK, Myers J. Immunohistochemical demonstration of chlamydial antigens in association with prostatitis. Mod Pathol 1988;1: 348–51.

[43] Ohkawa M, Yamaguchi K, Tokunaga S, et al. Ureaplasma urealyticum in the urogenital tract of patients with chronic prostatitis or related symptomatology. Br J Urol 1993;72:918–21.

[44] Potts JM, Sharma R, Pasqualotto F, et al. Association of Ureaplasma urealyticum with abnormal reactive oxygen species levels and absence of leukocytospermia. J Urol 2000;163:1775–8.

[45] Krieger JN, Riley DE. Prostatitis: what is the role of infection? Int J Antimicrob Agents 2002;19: 475–9.

[46] Schneider H, Ludwig M, Hossain HM, et al. The 2001 Giessen Cohort Study on patients with prostatitis syndrome: an evaluation of inflammatory status and search for microorganisms 10 years after a first analysis. Andrologia 2003;35:258–62.

[47] Soto SM, Smithson A, Martinez JA, et al. Biofilm formation in uropathogenic Escherichia coli strains: relationship with prostatitis, urovirulence factors and antimicrobial resistance. J Urol 2007; 177:365–8.

[48] Kanamaru S, Kurazono H, Terai A, et al. Increased biofilm formation in Escherichia coli isolated from acute prostatitis. Int J Antimicrob Agents 2006; 28S:S21–5.

[49] Johnson JR, Kuskowski MA, Gajewski A, et al. Extended virulence genotypes and phylogenetic background of Escherichia coli isolates from patients with cystitis, pyelonephritis, or prostatitis. J Infect Dis 2005;191:46–50.

[50] Costerton JW, Lewandowski Z, Caldwell DE, et al. Microbial biofilms. Annu Rev Microbiol 1995;49: 711–45.

[51] Costerton JW, Cheng K-J, Geesey GG. Bacterial biofilms in nature and disease. Annu Rev Microbiol 1987;41:435–64.

[52] Benson PJ, Smith CS. Cytomegalovirus prostatitis. Urology 1992;40:165–7.

[53] Hood SV, Bell D, McVey R, et al. Prostatitis and epididymo-orchitis due to Apergillus fumigatus in a patient with AIDS. Clin Infect Dis 1998;26: 229–31.

[54] Adams JR, Mata JA, Culkin DJ, et al. Acquired immune deficiency syndrome manifesting as prostate nodule secondary to cryptococcal infection. Urology 1992;39:289–91.

[55] Marans HY, Mandell W, Kislak JW, et al. Prostatic abscess due to histoplasma capsulatum in the acquired immune deficiency syndrome. J Urol 1991; 145:1275–6.

[56] Heyns CF, Fisher M. The urological management of the patient with acquired immunodeficiency syndrome. BJU Int 2005;95:709–16.

[57] Stamey TA, Meares EM, Winningham DG. Chronic bacterial prostatitis and the diffusion of drugs into prostatic fluid. J Urol 1970;103:187–94.

[58] Naber KG, Sorgel F. Antibiotic therapy: rationale and evidence for optimal drug concentrations in prostatic and seminal fluid and in prostatic tissue. Andrologia 2003;35:331–5.

[59] Butilla J, Kinzig-Schippers M, Naber CK, et al. Limitations in the use of drug cocktails (DC) to compare the pharmacokinetics (PK) of drugs: ciprofloxacin (CIP) vs. levofloxacin (LEV). Abstr Intersci Conf Antimicrob Agents Chemother Intersci Conf Antimicrob Agents Chemother 2000;40:18. Available at: http://gateway.nlm.nih.gov/MeetingAbstracts/1022 48598.html.

[60] Shoskes DA, Zeitlin SI. Use of prostatic massage in combination with antibiotics in the treatment of chronic prostatitis. Prostate Cancer Prostatic Dis 1999;2:159–63.

[61] Naber KG. Antibiotic treatment of chronic bacterial prostatitis. In: Nickel JC, editor. Textbook of prostatitis. Oxford (UK): Isis Medical Media Ltd.; 1999. p. 285–92.

[62] Nickel JC. α-Blockers for treatment of the prostatitis syndromes. Rev Urol 2005;7(8):S18–25.

[63] Moon TD. Alpha-blockers in prostatitis. Current Prostate Reports 2004;2:143–7.

[64] Barbalias GA, Nikiforidis G, Liatsikos EN. α-Blockers for the treatment of chronic prostatitis

in combination with antibiotics. J Urol 1998;159: 883–7.

[65] Alexander RB, Propert KJ, Schaeffer AJ, et al. Ciprofloxacin or tamsulosin in men with chronic prostatitis/chronic pelvic pain syndrome: a randomized, double-blind trial. Ann Intern Med 2004; 141(8):581–9.

[66] Hennenfent BR, Feliciano AE. Changes in white blood cell counts in men undergoing thrice-weekly prostatic massage, microbial diagnosis and antimicrobial therapy for genitourinary complaints. Br J Urol 1998;81:370–6.

[67] Keith IM, Jin J, Neal D Jr, et al. Cell relationship in a wistar rat model of spontaneous prostatitis. J Urol 2001;166:323–8.

[68] Kirby RS, Lowe D, Bultitude MI, et al. Intraprostatic urinary reflux: an aetiological factor in abacterial prostatitis. Br J Urol 1982;54: 729–31.

[69] Blacklock NJ. The anatomy of the prostate: relationship with prostatic infection. Infection 1991; 19(3):S111–4.

[70] Fayez A, Hani R, et al. Evaluation of prostatic massage in treatment of chronic prostatitis. Urology 2006;67(4):674–8.

[71] Nickel JC, Alexander R, Anderson R, et al. Prostatitis unplugged? Prostatic massage revisited. Tech Urol 1999;5(1):1–7.

[72] Difuccia B, Keith I, Teunissen B, et al. Diagnosis of prostatic inflammation: efficacy of needle biopsies versus tissue blocks. Urology 2005;65(3):445–8.

[73] Roberts RO, Bergstralh EJ, Bass SE, et al. Prostatitis as a risk factor for prostate cancer. Epidemiology 2004;15(1):93–9.

ELSEVIER
SAUNDERS

Urol Clin N Am 35 (2008) 33–46

UROLOGIC
CLINICS
of North America

Sexually Transmitted Infections

Tara Lee Frenkl, MD, MPH[a],*, Jeannette Potts, MD[b]

[a]Division of Urology, University of Pennsylvania, 3400 Civic Center Boulevard, 9 Penn Tower,
Philadelphia, PA 19104, USA
[b]Glickman Urological and Kidney Institute, Cleveland Clinic Foundation, 9500 Euclid Avenue,
A100, Cleveland, OH 44195, USA

Primary prevention through universal safe-sex precautions would eliminate the costly and sometimes tragic consequences of sexually transmitted infections (STI). However, because STI transmission remains prevalent, secondary prevention through screening and early diagnosis remains our most valuable weapon against the devastating disease sequelae. Early detection and appropriate antibiotic therapy have led to decreases in bacterial venereal diseases. For example, the incidence of syphilis in the United States has decreased from 51,000 in 1990 to 8,724 in 2005 [1]. Likewise, the incidence of gonorrhea has decreased from one million in 1980 to less than 340,000 cases documented in 2005 [2].

Chlamydia trachomatis remains the most common reportable bacterial STI, with an estimated 2.8 million new cases in the United States each year and 50 million worldwide [3]. Viral infections, for which curative therapy is not available, have been stable or increasing in prevalence. With 500,000 new cases each year, herpes simplex virus (HSV) is one of the most common viral STI. One million new cases of human papilloma virus are diagnosed each year, and the prevalence of this disease is between 24 and 40 million.

People at high risk of contracting sexually transmitted diseases are young adults between the ages of 18 and 28. The highest rate of gonorrhea and chlamydia infections is among

females age 15 to 19 [4]. It is also important to bear in mind that sexually transmitted diseases rank among the top five risks of international travelers, along with diarrhea, hepatitis, and motor vehicle accidents [5].

A urologist should have a high index of suspicion for underlying sexually transmitted disease in women who present with recurrent urinary-tract infections (UTIs) and in those who are symptomatic with sterile urine cultures. Up to 50% of women with signs of UTI during emergency department examination had subsequent positive cultures for sexually transmitted disease [6]. Physicians should maintain the same level of vigilance when treating women who have sex with women. Genital human papilloma virus has been identified along with squamous intraepithelial lesions among lesbians, and occurs among those who have not had sexual relations with men [7]. A high prevalence of bacterial vaginosis has been observed between monogamous lesbians. Because of more frequent orogenital practices, they may also be at higher risk of HSV type 1 [4].

Proctitis may occur in women and men who have anal sex. Causative organisms include *Neisseria gonorrhoeae*, *Chlamydia trachomatis*, *Treponema pallidum*, and HSV. A discussion of human immunodeficiency virus (HIV) is beyond the scope of this article; however, it is important to remember that STIs—especially the ulcerative types—facilitate the transmission and infection of HIV. HSV-2, in particular, may play a role in the transmission of HIV, as it has been identified more frequently than other STI among HIV-concordant couples [8].

The most common sexually transmitted diseases are discussed in this article. They include

Dr. Frenkl is an employee of Merck Research Labs as an Associate Director of Clinical Research in the area of Urology.

* Corresponding author.
E-mail address: tara_frenkl@merck.com
(T.L. Frenkl).

HSV, Chlamydia urethritis/cervicitis, lympho-granuloma venereum, syphilis, gonorrhea (GC), chancroid, trichomoniasis, and human papilloma virus (HPV). Other sexually associated pathogens which cause urethritis and vaginitides will also be discussed briefly.

Expedited partner therapy

A common dilemma for physicians treating patients with an STI is how to expeditiously extend treatment to the partner to both prevent complications from infection, such as pelvic inflammatory disease, and prevent the spread of disease. Traditional methods of patient or physician referral have obvious benefits and limitations. Expedited partner therapy (EPT) is the practice of treating the sexual partners of patients with STI by providing the patient with a prescription or medication to take to their partner without an intervening clinical evaluation or professional prevention counseling.

In August of 2006, the Centers for Disease Control (CDC) concluded that EPT has been shown to be at least equivalent to patient referral in preventing persistent or recurrent GC or chlamydial infection in heterosexuals and released guidelines for the uses of EPT [9]. The guidelines recommend that EPT should only be implemented when other management strategies are impractical or unsuccessful. All recipients should be encouraged to seek medical attention, in addition to accepting therapy by EPT, through counseling of the index case, written materials, and personal counseling by a pharmacist or other personnel. The CDC guidelines suggest that EPT may be used to treat GC and chlamydial infection in heterosexual women and men. It should not be used routinely in men who have sex with men (MSM) because of a lack of data to confirm efficacy in this population and the high risk of comorbidity, especially with undiagnosed HIV. Similarly, EPT should not be used for partners of women with trichomoniasis because of the high risk of comorbidity with chlamydia or GC. EPT is not recommended for routine use in the management of patients with infectious syphilis.

To address legal and medicolegal status of EPT, the CDC collaborated with the Center for Law and the Public's Health at Georgetown and Johns Hopkins Universities to assess the legal framework concerning EPT in all 50 states, the District of Columbia, and Puerto Rico. The objective of the research was to conceptualize and identify legal provisions that implicate a clinician's ability to execute EPT. Currently, EPT is allowable in 11 states, potentially allowable in 28 states, and legally prohibited in 13 states. The results of the research, explanation, and legal status for each state can be found at the CDC Web site http://www.cdc.gov/std/ept/legal/default.htm.

Genital ulcers

Several sexually transmitted infections are clinically characterized by the genital ulcers typically associated with them, most commonly HSV, syphilis, and chancroid. In 2002, it was estimated that over 45 million persons had HSV, while only 6,862 cases of syphilis, and 67 cases of chancroid were reported.

Although specificity for clinical diagnosis of genital ulcer disease is good (94%–98%), sensitivity is quite low (31%–35%) [10]. Inguinal lymph node findings did not contribute to diagnostic accuracy. Confirmatory cultures and serologic testing for syphilis, chancroid, and HSV should be performed whenever possible. Specifically, the CDC recommends: (1) serology and either darkfield examination or direct immunofluorescence for *T. pallidum*; (2) culture or antigen test for herpes simplex virus; and (3) culture for *H. ducreyi*. It should be kept in mind that patients may be coinfected with more than one sexually transmitted disease. Approximately 10% of patients with chancroid are coinfected with HSV or syphilis. HIV testing should be strongly considered in the management of patients with confirmed STI. Clinical characteristics of sexually transmitted genital ulcers are summarized in Table 1. Other causes that are not sexually transmitted, such as Behcet's syndrome, drug reaction, erythema multiforme, Crohn's disease, lichen planus, amebiasis, trauma, and carcinoma should also be considered in the differential diagnosis. Empiric treatment for the most likely cause based on history and physical should be initiated as laboratory test results are pending. If ulcers do not respond to therapy or appear unusual, a biopsy should be performed.

Herpes simplex virus

Diagnosis

Genital herpes infection is common, afflicting more than 50 million people in the United States. It is caused by herpes simplex virus type 2

Table 1
Genital ulcer disease

Disease	Lesions	Lymphadenopathy	Systemic symptoms
Primary syphillis	Painless, indurated, clean-based, usually singular	Nontender, rubbery, nonsuppurative bilateral lymphadenopathy	None
Genital herpes	Painful vesicles, shallow, usually multiple	Tender, bilateral inguinal adenopathy	Present during primary infection
Charncroid	Tender papule, then painful, undermined purulent ulcer, single or multiple	Tender, regional, painful, suppurative nodes	None
Lympho-granuloma	Small, painless vesical or papule progresses to an ulcer	Painful, matted, large nodes, develop with fistula tracts	Present after genital lesion heals

(HSV-2) in 85% to 90% of cases and herpes simplex virus type 1 (HSV-1) in 10% to 15% of cases. HSV-1 is responsible for common cold sores but can be transmitted via oral secretions during oral-genital sex. Silent infection is common and may account for more than 75% of viral transmission [11]. Up to 80% of women with HSV-2 antibodies have no history of clinical infection [12]. The incubation period ranges from 1 to 26 days but is usually short, approximately 4 days. Nongenital infection of HSV-1 during childhood may be protective to some extent against subsequent genital HSV-2 infection in adults. When exposed to HSV-2, women with negative HSV-1 antibodies had a 32% risk of infection per year, whereas women with positive antibodies had a 10% risk of infection per year.

Primary infection manifests with painful ulcers of the genitalia or anus, and bilateral painful inguinal adenopathy. The initial presentation for HSV-1 and HSV-2 are the same, though HSV-1 is expected to become the more common cause of first episode [4]. A group of vesicles on an erythematous base that does not follow a neural distribution is pathognomonic for herpes simplex [13].

The initial infection is often associated with constitutional flu-like symptoms. Sacral radiculomyelopathy is a rare manifestation of primary infection that has a greater association with primary anal HSV. Genital lesions, especially urethral lesions, may cause transient urinary retention in women. Recurrent episodes are usually less severe, involving only ulceration of the genital or anal area. Severe disease and complications of herpes include pneumonitis, disseminated infection, hepatitis, meningitis, and encephalitis. Asymptomatic shedding occurs more frequently with HSV-2 than HSV-1, even in patients with long standing or clinically silent infection. Asymptomatic viral shedding is more likely during the 3- to 12-month period following clinical presentation, thereby perpetuating the risk of transmission [4,13].

The diagnosis of genital herpes should not be made on clinical suspicion alone, as the classic presentation of the ulcer occurs in only a small percentage of patients. Women especially, may present with atypical lesions such as abrasions, fissures, or itching [14]. Viral culture with subtyping has been the gold standard of diagnosis of herpes infection. The viral subtype should be determined in every patient, as it is important for prognosis and counseling. Women with HSV-2 have an average of four recurrences within the first year and women with HSV-1 have one recurrence in the first year. After the first year, HSV-1 rarely recurs while the rate of HSV-2 decreases, but slowly [15]. Viral culture can generally isolate the virus in 5 days, is relatively inexpensive, and highly specific. However, the sensitivity of viral culture ranges from 30% to 95%, depending on the stage of the lesion and whether it is the primary infection or a recurrence. Viral load is highest when the lesion is vesicular and during primary infection. Therefore viral culture has the highest sensitivity at these times and declines sharply as the lesion heals.

There are currently four Food and Drug Administration (FDA) approved glycoprotein G-based type-specific antibody assays that identify antibodies to HSV glycoproteins G-1 and G-2, which evoke a type-specific antibody response [16]. These tests may also be able to identify recently acquired versus established HSV infection based on antibody avidity [17]. Point-of-care tests can provide results for HSV-2 antibodies from capillary blood or serum during a clinic visit [2].

Treatment

Antiviral therapies approved for treatment include oral acyclovir, valacyclovir, and famciclovir. Recommended antiviral regimens are listed in Table 2. Topical antiviral medications are not effective. Recurrences can be treated with an episodic or suppressive approach. When used for episodic treatment, medication must be initiated during the prodrome or within 1 day of the onset of lesions. Daily suppressive therapy has been shown to prevent 80% of recurrences and is an option for patients who suffer from frequent recurrences. It has been shown to decrease the frequency and duration of recurrences as well as viral shedding, and therefore reduction in the rate of transmission. The safety and efficacy of daily suppressive therapy has been well documented.

Chancroid

Diagnosis

Chancroid, caused by *Haemophilus ducreyi,* is the most common STI worldwide. It affects men three times more often than women. The incubation period ranges from 1 to 21 days. It causes a painful, nonindurated ulcer on the penis or vulvovaginal area. The ulcer has a friable base covered with a gray or yellow purulent exudate and a shaggy border. It can spread laterally by apposition to inner thighs and buttocks, especially in women. It is associated with inguinal adenopathy that is typically unilateral and tender, with tendency to be become suppurative and fistulize.

Haemophilus ducreyi is fastidious and difficult to culture. The special culture media is not widely available and sensitivity of culture remains under 80%. Gram-stain of a specimen obtained from the undermined edge of the ulcer may be more helpful in identifying the short, fine, Gram-negative streptobacilli, which are usually arranged in short, parallel chains. Recently, polymerase chain reaction (PCR) assays have been shown to be a sensitive and specific means of detecting *Haemophilus ducreyi.* Although no PCR test is currently FDA approved, testing can be performed by commercial agencies. Approximately 10% of persons who have chancroid are coinfected with *T. pallidum* or HSV [2]. HIV and syphilis screening should be performed at the time of diagnosis and 3 months after treatment, if initially negative.

Four criteria should be considered in formulating the diagnosis of chancroid: presence of one or more painful ulcers, presence of regional lymphadenopathy, a negative T pallidum evaluation or negative serologies at least 7 days after the onset of symptoms, and negative HSV culture from the ulcer exudates [4].

Treatment

Single dose treatments consist of azithromycin, 1 g orally or ceftriaxone, 250 mg intramuscularly. Alternative regimens include ciprofloxacin, 500 mg twice daily for 3 days, or erythromycin base, 500 mg by mouth three times daily for 7 days; however, antibiotic susceptibility varies geographically. Resistance has been reported to ciprofloxacin and erythromycin in some regions. Ciprofloxacin is contraindicated during pregnancy and lactation. Subjective improvement should be noted within 3 days and ulcers generally heal completely in 7 to 14 days. Healing may be slower in uncircumcised men with ulcers below the foreskin and in patients with HIV [18]. Patients should be re-examined in 5 to 7 days. Sexual partners should be examined and treated if sexual relations were held within 2 weeks before or during the eruption

Table 2
Recommended oral treatment for genital HSV

Agent	First clinical episode	Episodic therapy	Suppressive therapy
Acyclovir	400 mg tid for 7–10 days or 200 mg 5 times/day for 7–10 days	400 mg tid for 5 days or 200 mg 5 times/day for 5 days or 800 mg bid for 5 days	400 mg bid
Famiciclovir	250 mg tid for 7–10 days	125 mg bid for 5 days	250 mg bid
Valacyclovir	1 g bid for 7–10 days	500 mg bid for 3–5 days or 1 g qd for 5 days	500 mg qd or 1 g qd

Data from Centers for Disease Control and Prevention. Sexually Transmitted Diseases Guidelines 2002. MMWR 2002;51(RR06):1–80.

of the ulcer. Symptomatic relief of inguinal tenderness can be provided by needle aspiration or incision and drainage of the buboes.

Syphilis

Diagnosis

Syphilis is caused by a spirochete, *Treponema pallidum*. Incubation periods range between 10 and 90 days. It is spread through contact with infectious lesions or body fluids. It can also be acquired in utero and through blood transfusion. Primary syphilis is characterized by a single painless, indurated ulcer occurring at the site of inoculation, that appears about 3 weeks after inoculation and persists for 4 to 6 weeks. The ulcer is typically found on the glans, corona, or perianal area on men and on the labial or anal area on women. It is often associated with bilateral, nontender inguinal or regional lymphadenopathy. Since the ulcer and adenopathy are painless and heal without treatment, primary syphilis often goes unnoticed.

Latent syphilis is defined as seroreactivity with no clinical evidence of disease. Early latent syphilis is latent syphilis acquired within the past year. All other latent syphilis is either referred to as late latent syphilis or latent syphilis of unknown duration.

Secondary syphilis usually begins 4 to 10 weeks after the appearance of the ulcer, but may present as long as 24 months following the initial infection. Secondary syphilis manifests with mucocutaneous, constitutional, and parenchymal signs and symptoms. Frequent early manifestations consist of maculopapular rash, which is commonly seen on the trunk and arms, and generalized nontender lymphadenopathy. After several days or weeks, a papular rash may accompany the primary rash. These papular lesions are associated with endarteritis and may therefore become necrotic and pustular. The distribution widens and commonly affects the palms and soles. In the intertriginous areas, these papules may enlarge and erode to produce condyloma lata, which are particularly infectious. Less common manifestations of secondary syphilis include hepatitis and immune complex-induced glomerulonephritis.

Approximately one third of untreated patients will develop tertiary syphilis. It is very rare in industrialized countries, except for occasional cases reported in HIV patients. Syphilis is a systemic disease that can affect almost any organ or system, especially the cardiovascular, skeletal, and central nervous systems, and skin. Aortitis, meningitis, uveitis, optic neuritis, general paresis, tabe dorsalis, and gummas of the skin and skeleton are just some of the sequalae associated with tertiary syphilis.

Dark-field microscopy and direct fluorescent antibody (DFA) are tests of specimens obtained from primary or secondary lesions. Dark field microscopy is not widely available but DFA testing of a fixed smear from a lesion can be performed at many commercial laboratories. Nontreponemal serologic testing, with rapid plasma regain (RPR) or venereal disease research laboratory (VRDL) are the most common methods of screening suspected individuals. Sensitivity is 78% and 86% for RPR and VDRL, respectively, in primary syphilis, 100% for both in secondary syphilis, and over 95% in tertiary syphilis [19]. The false positive rate is approximately 1% to 2% and may be secondary to a large variety of causes [20]. Therefore, all positive tests should be confirmed with treponemal testing using *T. pallidum* particle agglutination or florescent treponemal antibody absorbed. HIV can cause false negative results by both treponemal and nontreponemal methods [21,22]. Positive treponemal antibody tests usually remain positive for life and do not correlate with disease activity. Nontreponemal antibody titers, RPR and VDRL, correlate with disease activity. These tests usually become negative 1 year after treatment. For following disease activity, the same test, either RPR or VRDL, should be performed at the same lab, as the results are not interchangeable and may vary from laboratory to laboratory.

The United States Preventive Services Task Force recommends that pregnant women and people who are at higher risk for syphilis infection receive screening tests for the disease [23]. People at higher risk for syphilis include men who have sex with men and engage in high-risk sexual behavior, commercial sex workers, persons who exchange sex for drugs, and those in adult correctional facilities. The CDC recommends that HIV testing should be considered in the initial evaluation of all patients with syphilitic infection, and that screening for hepatitis B and C, gonorrhea, and chlamydial infection also should be considered. The presence of chancres increases the risk of HIV acquisition two to five fold [24,25].

Treatment

Benzthiazide penicillin G (2.4 million units intramuscularly as a single dose) remains the treatment of choice. Other parental preparations or oral penicillin are not acceptable substitutes. The Jarisch-Herxheimer reaction is a reaction consisting of headache, myalgia, fever, tachycardia, and increased respiratory rate that occur within the first 24 hours after treatment with penicillin. Patients should be warned about the reaction and it is usually managed with bed rest and nonsteroidal anti-inflammatory agents. It may cause fetal distress and preterm labor in pregnant women.

If the patient has penicillin allergy, doxycycline 100 mg by mouth twice daily or tetracycline 500 mg four times daily for 14 days, are accepted alternatives. Ceftriaxone 1 gram IM or IV daily for 8–10 days has also been recommended by some specialists. For late latent syphilis, latent syphilis of unknown duration, or tertiary syphilis, benzthiazide penicillin injection of 2.4 million units should be repeated weekly for a total of three doses, or doxycycline or tetracycline therapy extended for a total of 4 weeks. Doxycycline and tetracycline are contraindicated in pregnancy. Therefore desensitization to penicillin is recommended if a pregnant patient has a penicillin allergy.

Neurosyphilis is treated with aqueous crystalline penicillin G, 3 to 4 million units intravenously every 4 hours for 10 to 14 days; or penicillin G procaine, 2.4 million units intramuscularly (IM) once daily, plus probenecid, 500 mg orally four times daily, with both drugs given for 10 to 14 days. Probenecid cannot be used in patients with an allergy to sulfa. Patients should be followed with nontreponemal antibody titers at 6 and 12 months. Patients with neurosyphilis require repeat examination of cerebrospinal fluid 3 to 6 months following therapy and every 6 months afterwards until normal results are achieved.

Lymphogranuloma venereum

Diagnosis

Lymphogranuloma venereum is caused by *Chlamydia trachomatis* types L1, L2, and L3, and is extremely rare in the United States. It still persists in parts of Africa, Asia, South America, and the Caribbean [26]. The incubation period ranges from 3 to 30 days. The initial manifestation of infection is usually a single, painless ulcer on the penis, anus, or vulvovaginal area that goes unnoticed. Patients usually present with painful unilateral suppurative inguinal adenopathy and constitutional symptoms that occur 2 to 6 weeks

after resolution of the ulcer. Women and homosexual men may present with proctocolitis and perirectal or deep iliac lymph-node enlargement if the primary lesion arises from the rectum or cervix. Significant tissue injury and scarring may occur, leading to labial fenestration, urethral destruction, anorectal fistulas, and elephantiasis of the penis, scrotum, or labia.

The diagnosis is mainly clinical and cultures are positive in only 30% to 50% of cases. Compliment-fixation or indirect-fluorescence antibody titers can confirm diagnosis. A compliment fixation titer greater or equal to 64 is diagnostic of infection. Other causes of inguinal adenopathy should be excluded.

Treatment

Antibiotic therapy for 3 weeks is necessary, using either doxycycline, 100 mg twice daily or erythromycin, 500 mg four times daily. Doxycycline is contraindicated in pregnant and lactating women. Patients should be followed clinically until symptoms resolve. Sexual partners should be examined, tested for urethral or cervical infection, and treated if sexual relations were held within 30 days of the onset of symptoms.

Buboes may require aspiration or incision and drainage to prevent femoral or inguinal ulcerations. Azithromycin, 1 g by mouth weekly for 3 weeks may be a potential alternative for treatment, but data is still lacking.

Urethritis, epididymitis, and cervicitis

Diagnosis of urethritis in men is based on any one of the following three criteria: mucopurulent or purulent penile discharge, Gram stain of urethral secretions demonstrating more than 5 white blood cells (WBC) per oil immersion field, or positive leukocyte esterase on first-void urine (or first-void urine specimen demonstrating more than 10 WBC per oil immersion field). Gonococcal urethritis can be diagnosed by Gram stain, as a positive Gram stain is 99% specific and 95% sensitive. However, a negative Gram stain in the setting of urethritis, does not rule out gonococcus [4].

Epididymitis is defined as inflammation of the epididymis and may be infectious (bacterial, viral, fungal, or parasitic) or noninfectious (trauma, autoimmune, amiodarone-induced). The differential diagnosis of testicular torsion must also be considered, as this is a surgical emergency that could result in testicular loss if not treated immediately. In young men, the most common cause of infectious epididymitis is sexually transmitted infection. In heterosexual men less than 35 years old, the most common causes are *N. gonorrhoeae* and *C. trachomatis*. In MSM, *E coli* and *Haemophilus influenzae* are the most common [27].

Patients usually present with scrotal swelling and pain. Palpation may reveal a prominent and tender epididymis or a large tense erythematous mass, which is painful and warm to touch. If it also involves the testis it is known as epididymo-orchitis. Laboratory findings that are consistent with a diagnosis of epididymitis include pyuria, bacteriuria, a positive urine culture, and leukocytosis; however, normal urinalysis and white count do not rule it out. The CDC recommends that the evaluation of men for epididymitis should include one of the following: Gram stain of urethral secretions demonstrating more 5 WBC per oil immersion field (gonococcal infection is established by documenting the presence of WBC containing intracellular Gram-negative diplococci on urethral Gram stain) or positive leukocyte esterase test or pyuria (more than 10 WBC per high power field) on first-void urine. Culture, nucleic acid hybridization tests, and nucleic acid amplification tests previously discussed for gonorrhea and chlamydia should be performed. For patients at risk, consideration should be given for further sexually transmitted disease (STD) testing. Treatment includes supportive therapy of bed rest, scrotal elevation, anti-inflammatory agents and ceftriaxone, 250 mg IM in a single dose plus doxycycline, 100 mg orally twice a day for 10 days. For epididymitis most likely caused by enteric organisms, or for patients allergic to cephalosporins or tetracyclines, treatment should include ofloxacin, 300 mg orally twice a day for 10 days, or levofloxacin, 500 mg orally once daily for 10 days. In an acute setting, testicular torsion should be an important consideration in the differential diagnosis.

Cervicitis is characterized by two major diagnostics signs: purulent or mucopurulent endocervical exudate or sustained endocervical bleeding, easily provoked by swabbing the cervical os. Indeed, some women with cervicitis may have no other symptoms than bleeding post coitally or abnormal vaginal discharge.

The following sections address the most common causes of cervicitis, urethritis, and epididymitis in patients with STD exposure.

Chlamydia trachomatis

Diagnosis

Chalmydia trachomatis is the most common bacterial STD in the United States and the most common worldwide. In the United States it is most prevalent in sexually active adolescents and young adults. Virulent serotypes include D, E, F, G, H, I, J, and K. The incubation period ranges from 3 to 14 days.

The majority of both of men and women are asymptomatic. Approximately 50% of men experience lower urinary-tract symptoms attributed to urethritis, epididymitis, or prostatitis, and may notice clear or white urethral discharge. *C. trachomatis* is the most common cause of epididymitis in young men. Approximately 75% of women are asymptomatic and 40% with untreated infection will develop pelvic inflammatory disease (PID) [28]. Scarring of the fallopian tubes from chlamydial infection puts patients at risk for recurrent PID with vaginal flora, ectopic pregnancy, pelvic pain, and infertility [29]. Chlamydia may also be transmitted to newborns during vaginal birth through exposure of the mother's infected cervix. Neonates may contract ocular, oropharygeal, respiratory, urogenital, or rectal infection.

Selective screening has been shown to reduce the incidence of PID [30]. Women should be screened annually until age 25, or if risk factors such as a new sexual partner are present. In women, screening may be accomplished by: (1) A nucleic acid amplification test (NAAT) performed on an endocervical swab specimen, if a pelvic examination is acceptable; otherwise, a NAAT performed on urine; (2) an unamplified nucleic acid hybridization test, an enzyme immunoassay, or direct fluorescent antibody test performed on an endocervical swab specimen; or 3) culture performed on an endocervical swab specimen. In men, the options remain the same but intraurethral samples must be used.

Treatment

Azithromycin, 1 g by mouth as a single dose, or doxycycline, 100 mg twice daily for 7 days, are primary treatments and equally effective. Alternative therapies include erythromycin base, 500 mg four times daily, erythromycin ethylsuccinate, 800 mg four times daily, ofloxacin, 300 mg twice daily, or levofloxacin, 500 mg daily for 7 days. Doxycycline, erythromycin estolate, and ofloxacin are contraindicated during pregnancy.

Erythromycin base, erythromycin ethylsuccinate, and azithromycin are safe during pregnancy. Another alternative in pregnant women includes amoxicillin, 500 mg three times per day for 7 days. Partners should be examined, tested, and treated. Patients should refrain from sexual intercourse until both their and their partner's treatment is completed, or 7 days after single dose therapy. Reculture for cure is not needed for patients treated with doxycycline or a quinolone antibiotic. It is recommended 3 weeks after treatment with erythromycin, as cure rates are lower with this regimen, in pregnant women, or if the patient has persistent symptoms. However, patients with chlamydia are at high risk for reinfection and should be rescreened 3 to 4 months after treatment.

Gonorrhea

Diagnosis

Gonorrhea is caused by a Gram-negative diplococcus, *Neisseria gonorrhoeae*. The incubation period ranges from 3 to 14 days. Risk of infection after one exposure is 10% in men and 40% in women. Men will usually experience lower urinary-tract symptoms attributed to urethritis, epididymitis, proctitis, or prostatitis, with associated mucopurulent urethral discharge. Women may have symptoms of vaginal and pelvic discomfort, dysuria, or abnormal vaginal discharge, but are most often asymptomatic. Both symptomatic and asymptomatic infections can lead to PID and its subsequent complications. Therefore, screening in all sexually active adolescents and women up to the age of 25 should be performed yearly. In addition, any women with risk factors, such as a new sexual partner or multiple sexual partners, should be screened. Manifestations of gonococcal dissemination are rare today and include arthritis, dermatitis, meningitis, and endocarditis.

The CDC recommends screening by culture on an endocervical swab specimen in women or an intraurethral swab in men [31]. A positive Gram stain of a male urethral swab is highly specific (99%) and sensitive (95%). Presence of WBC and diplococci are confirmatory; however a negative Gram stain does not rule out GC. Gram stain of secretions from pharynx, cervix, or rectum are insufficient for the diagnosis of GC and are not recommended [4]. Culture and sensitivity are important to monitor antibiotic susceptibility

and resistance. Culture may be performed on urethra exudates if present. If transport and storage conditions are not conducive to maintaining the viability of *N. gonorrhoeae*, a NAAT or nucleic acid hybridization test can be performed. If it is not possible to obtain an intraurethral or edocervical specimen, NAAT may be performed on urine. Urine NAATs for *N. gonorrhoeae* have been shown to be less sensitive than endocervial and intraurethral swabs in astympotomatic men [32].

Treatment

The most highly recommended treatment for gonorrhea is ceftriaxone, 125 mg IM as a single dose. It produces high, sustained blood levels that result in cure in over 99% of uncomplicated cases at all anatomic sites. An oral alternative is a single oral dose of cefixime, 400 mg. Cefixime is no longer available in tablet formulation in the United States but can be obtained as a suspension. Alternative single-dose parenteral agents for urogenital and anorectal gonorrhea include ceftizoxime 500 mg IM, cefoxitin 2 g IM with probenecid, 1 g orally, or cefotaxime 500 mg IM. For patients with penicillin or cephalosporin allergies, a single intramuscular dose of spectinomycin, 2 g is a recommended alternative but not available in the United States. A single oral 2-g dose of azithromycin is effective in uncomplicated infections, but is not recommended by the CDC because of increasing resistance. It may be an option for treatment of uncomplicated infections in patients with documented severe allergic reactions to penicillins or cephalosporins.

Over the past decade, there has been the rapid emergence of quinolone-resistant *N.gonorrhoeae* (QRNG). Areas where QRNG are most prevalent include parts of Asia, the Pacific, Hawaii, and California [33]. Initially, quinolones were not advised as primary therapy in these states or in patients who have had recent sexual encounters with people from these areas. However, quinolone resistance in other areas in the United States has rapidly increased. In April 2007, the CDC announced that it no longer recommends quinolones for the treatment of gonoccocal infection in any population. Quinolones are contraindicated during pregnancy. Spectinomycin, 2 g IM can be used during pregnancy or in patients allergic to quinolones and cephalosporins. Spectinomycin is not as effective for pharyngeal infection.

Patients infected with gonorrhea are often coinfected with *C. trachomatis*. It has been recommended that patients undergo simultaneous dual treatment because the cost of treatment is less than that of chlamydial testing. All patients with diagnosed with gonorrhea should be treated with for possible coinfection with *Chlamydia trachomatis* with a single dose of azithromycin, 1 g or with doxycycline, 100 mg twice a day for 7 days, unless chlamydial infection has been ruled out.

If more than 60 days has past, the most recent sexual partner should be evaluated and treated. Sexual activity should be avoided until both partners complete treatment and are symptom free. Persons with persistent symptoms or recurrence shortly after treatment should be reevaluated by culture for *N. gonorrhoeae* and positive isolates should undergo antimicrobial-susceptibility testing. Clinicians and laboratories should report treatment failures or resistant gonococcal isolates to the CDC at 404-639-8373 through state and local public health authorities [34].

Trichomoniasis

Diagnosis

Trichomonasis is one of the most common sexually transmitted diseases, with approximately 174 million new cases reported world-wide each year, and more than 8 million new cases reported yearly in North America [35]. There is an increased incidence in developing countries and in women who have had multiple sexual partners. It is caused by the flagellated protozoan *Trichomonas vaginalis*, which can inhabit the vagina, urethra, Bartholian glands, Skene's glands, and prostate. It cannot infect the rectum or mouth. The human being is its only known host. The incubation period ranges from 4 to 28 days.

Trichomoniasis is typically asymptomatic in men but may produce short-lived symptoms of urethral discharge, dysuria, and urinary urgency. Fifty percent of women are asymptomatic. Clinical manifestations in women include the sudden onset of a frothy white or green, foul smelling vaginal discharge, pruritis, and erythema. Other symptoms include dyspareunia, suprapubic discomfort, and urinary urgency. It has been associated with premature labor in pregnant women and with increased risk of HIV transmission [36,37].

Clinical examination may reveal a frothy discharge and the characteristic "strawberry vulva" or "strawberry cervix." However, clinical assessment alone is not specific enough for diagnosis. Typically, the vaginal discharge has an elevated pH. The motile protazoa, which are one to four times the size of polymorphonuclear cells, can also be seen on vaginal wet-mount smear or microscopic examination of urine (preferably voiding bottle #1). Microscopic inspection of vaginal secretions has only a 60% to 70% sensitivity [4]. In men the diagnosis is made with urethral culture or microscopic examination of urine (preferably voiding bottle #1). Standard culture, transport culture kits, enzyme immunoassay, nucleic acid amplification, and immunofluorescence techniques are also available for confirmatory testing.

Treatment

Infected individuals and their sexual partners should be treated to prevent recurrence of infection. A single 2-g dose of metronidazole is effective in most cases and can be used in the second trimester of pregnancy. Metronidazole therapy is associated with a 90% to 95% cure rate, while tinidazole 2-g single dose is associated with an 86% to 100% cure rate [4]. For nonpregnant treatment failures a longer course of metronidazole, 500 mg twice daily for 7 days, is recommended. The dosing regimens appear equally effective; however, side effects, especially gastrointestinal side effects, are more common with the high dose single therapy. Patients must abstain from alcohol consumption during therapy. Repeat testing at 5 to 7 days and 30 days should be performed if symptoms fail to resolve and treatment failure is suspected. A course of metronidazole, 500 mg twice a day for 7 days should be repeated, or 2 g once a day for 3 to 5 days may be tried. Metronidazole gel for intravaginal application is available; however, it is less than 50% effective as oral treatment.

Overview of other vaginitides

Ureaplasma urealyticum, *Mycoplasma hominis*, and *Mycoplasma genitalium* are considered commensal organisms of the genital tract in both men and women. It is estimated that at least 60% of sexually active women may harbor *Ureaplasma* in their genital tracts. These organisms however, have been implicated in cases of chronic prostatitis in men, urgency-frequency symptoms in women, [38] and in up to 40% of nongonococcal urethritis cases [39]. Currently, the initial recommended therapy is doxycycline, 100 mg twice daily for two weeks or a single dose of azythromycin, 1 g by mouth, which can be repeated in 10 to 14 days. Other alternatives include arithromyocine, 500 mg 4 times daily, or ofloxacin, 300 mg twice daily for 10 to 14 days. Sexual partners should be evaluated and treated accordingly.

Bacterial vaginosis (BV) is caused by the overgrowth of a *Gardnerella vaginalis*, anaerobic organisms, *Mycoplasma*, or the inhibition of normal vaginal flora. The cause for disruption of the microflora may be caused by douching, abnormal uterine bleeding, contraceptive use, or increased number of sexual partners. Vaginal secretions should be examined using 10% potassium hydroxide (KOH), to observe a fishy odor secondary to the release of amines. These specimens should also be examined under the microscope. Three out of the four following factors must be met to confirm the diagnosis of BV: (1) thin, white vaginal discharge that covers the vagina, (2) vaginal PH greater than 4.5, (3) clue cells, and (4) positive width test (KOH). There are commercially available DNA probes and card tests which can be used for office diagnosis. The recommended primary therapy includes metronidazole, 500 mg twice daily for 7 days, clindamycin cream 2% intravaginally at bedtime for 7 days, or metronidazole gel 0.75% intravaginally at bedtime for 5 days [40,41].

Vaginitis caused by *Candida albicans* is the most common type seen in the clinical setting; however, there are other species of *Candida* that may cause similar presentations. Characteristically, thick, cheesy vaginal discharge is usually associated with vulvar irritation and itching. However, patients may also experience vaginal discomfort, burning, dyspareunia, and external dysuria. The diagnosis can be confirmed in a woman with signs and symptoms by findings of yeast or psuedohyphae on a wet preparation slide, or a Gram stain of the vaginal discharge. The yeast and pseudohyphae are better seen after the application of 10% KOH. Over-the-counter antifungal vaginal creams, tablets, or suppositories of the topical azole class are generally effective and require 1 to 7 days of treatment. The treatment agents include butoconazole, clotrimazole, miconazole, and terconazole. An alternative to vaginal creams that is both effective and economical is fluconazole, 150 mg as a single oral dose. Recurrent infections should prompt evaluation to rule out diabetes mellitus and HIV.

Human papilloma virus

Diagnosis

Genital warts (*Condylomata acuminata*) are caused by human papilloma virus (HPV). HPV is a DNA-containing virus, which is spread by direct skin to skin contact. Over 100 types of HPV exist and over 30 types can infect the genital area. Risk factors for acquiring HPV include multiple sexual partners, early age on onset of sexual intercourse, and having a sexual partner with HPV. Most infections are subclinical and asymptomatic. It has been shown that 60% of a group of female college students followed by Papanikolaou (PAP) smear every 6 months for 3 years were infected with HPV at some point. The median duration of HPV infection was 8 months, with only 9% remaining infected after 2 years [42].

Types 6 and 11 of HPV are most often responsible for visible external genital warts. Patients may be infected with more than one type of HPV. Genital warts may appear anywhere on the external genitalia. It has been suggested that inoculation occurs at the site of genital microtrauma [43]. HPV has can also been found on the cervix, vagina, urethra, anus, and on mucous membranes such as the conjunctiva, mouth, and nasal passages.

Types 6 and 11 HPV are low risk for conversion to invasive carcinoma of the external genitalia. Some other types present in the anogenital region, notably types 16, 18, 31, 33, 35, 39, 45, and 51, have been associated with cervical dysplasia and neoplasm in women and squamous intraepithelial neoplasia in men [44–46]. Over 99% of cervical cancers and 84% of anal cancers are associated with HPV, most commonly HPV 16 and 18 [47,48]. Because HPV progresses rapidly in HIV-infected women, cervical cancer is considered one of the AIDS-defining illnesses. Smoking may increase the risk of dysplastic progression and malignancy in both men and women.

In women, HPV may be associated with non-specific symptoms, such as vulvodynia or pruritis. Malodorous vaginal discharge may also be a presenting sign, and the high rate of coinfection with other STDs observed in this setting may be a contributing factor.

The diagnosis is usually made through the visualization or palpation of nontender papillomatous genital lesions. Aceto-whitening with 3% to 5% acetic acid placed on a towel and wrapped around the genitals may show subclinical, flat condylomas appearing as whitish areas. Using this method, it was shown that 50% to 77% of steady male partners of women with HPV infection or cervical neoplasia had subclinical HPV infection [49]. Conversely, female partners of men with genital warts have a high incidence of HPV infection [50]. The benefit of evaluating and treating asymptomatic sexual partners of women with genital warts or abnormal PAP smears remains unclear. Routine androscopy is not recommended. Biopsies of genital warts are not routinely needed but should be undertaken in all instances of atypical, pigmented, indurated, fixed, or ulcerated warts. In addition, biopsy should be performed if the lesions persist or worsen after treatment, and in immunocompromised patients.

Treatment

The CDC currently recommends that patients with genital warts be informed that HPV and recurrence is common among sexual active persons, the incubation period can be long and variable, and duration of infection and methods of prevention are not definitively known. The choice of therapy for genital warts depends on several factors, including wart size, number and location, and patient and physician preference. Since genital warts spontaneously resolve with time, observation remains an option. Therapy can be patient applied or provider applied. Patient-applied therapies are less expensive and may be more effective than provider-applied therapy [51,52].

Recommended treatment choices for patient-applied therapy include podofilox 0.5% solution or gel and imiquimod 5% cream [53]. Podofilox solution should be applied every 12 hours for 3 days, then off for 4 days, with the option to repeat the treatment cycle four times. The total volume of solution used should not exceed 0.5 mL per day and the total wart area should not be greater than 10 cm^2. It may be helpful to demonstrate the first application in the office. Imiquimod cream should be applied three times per week at bedtime for up to 16 weeks. The area should be thoroughly washed 6 to 10 hours after application. Imiquimod should not be used on vaginal lesions as it has been reported to cause chronic ulceration. Neither medication should be used in pregnancy.

Options for provider-applied therapy include cryotherapy with liquid nitrogen, electrosurgery, laser therapy, podophyllin resin 20% to 25%,

trichloroacetic acid (TCA) or bichloroacateic acid (BCA) 80% to 90%, or surgical excision. Surgical excision may be accomplished by electorcautery or sharply with a tangential incision. Bleeding can generally be controlled with electorcautery or silver nitrate application. Surgical therapies appear to be equally effective with regards to clearance rates [54]. The advantages of surgical excision are that large warts or large areas can be addressed at one time. Carbon dioxide laser therapy is an alternative option for treatment.

Podophyllin 10% to 25% in compound tincture of benzoin is applied once and washed thoroughly 1 to 4 hours after treatment. To avoid possible complications associated with systemic absorption and toxicity of podophyllin, it is important to follow 2 guidelines: 1) application should be limited to <0.5 mL of podophyllin or an area of <10 cm^2 of warts per session, and 2) no open lesions or wounds should exist in the treatment area. Treatment may be repeated weekly as needed. Podophyllin is contraindicated during pregnancy. TCA and BCA should be carefully applied with a cotton tip applicator only to the warts at 1 to 2 week intervals. Patients will complain of a burning sensation that should resolve in 2 to 5 minutes. Unreacted acid should be removed with baking soda or talc. TCA and BCA are not preferable for keratinized or large warts. TCA is not absorbed and may be used during pregnancy.

Women with genital warts or a history of exposure should seek prompt gynecologic evaluation of the vagina and cervix. In the past, extensive vulvar lesions were treated with 5-fluorouracil (FU) cream, but it was reported to cause ulceration and acquired adenosis and its use is no longer recommended.

The presence of genital warts is not an indication for HPV testing, a change or frequency of PAP tests, or cervical colposcopy. HPV testing is not indicated for partners of persons with genital warts [4]. All patients however, should be reminded of the importance of regularly scheduled gynecologic exams and annual PAP tests.

Large or extensive lesions surrounding the meatus may herald the presence of urethral or bladder condyloma, warranting cystourethroscopy. Urethral or bladder lesions should be cystoscopically excised. Intraurethral 5% FU cream used twice weekly may be useful; however, it is limited by the great amount of inflammation produced [55]. Topical application of viable Bacille Calmette-Guerin has also shown promising preliminary results but larger studies are needed to fully evaluate its safety and efficacy [56].

HPV vaccine

Two virus-like particle HPV vaccines have been developed. One is a quadrivalent vaccine against HPV types 6, 11, 16, and 18 and was approved by the FDA in June 2006 for the prevention of HPV-associated conditions, such as cervical cancer, cervical cancer precursors, and anogenital warts. The other is a bivalent vaccine against HPV types 16 and 18 has been filed for FDA approval. The bivalent vaccine has been approved for use in Europe in September 2007. The surrogate marker for cervical cancer used in the clinical trials was the combined incidence of HPV 16- and 18-related grade 2 or 3 cervical intraepithelial neoplasia (CIN 2/3) or adenocarcinoma in situ (AIS) [57]. In study participants with no evidence of previous infection with the HPV 6, 11, 16, or 18, who completed the three immunization series with no protocol violations, the quadrivalent HPV vaccine showed 100% efficacy for preventing vaccine type-related CIN 2/3 and AIS, external genital warts, and vulval/vaginal intraepithelial neoplasia [58–60]. The vaccines also had high efficacy for the prevention of vaccine type HPV related persistent infection. Participants infected with one or more vaccine HPV types before vaccination were protected against disease caused by the remaining vaccine HPV types [61]. No evidence exists that the vaccines protect against disease caused by nonvaccine HPV types or for disease caused by vaccine types for which participants were PCR positive at baseline [57]. The bivalent vaccine also showed 100% efficacy in preventing HPV 16- or HPV 18-related CIN [62].

A subset of subjects in the phase II study of the quadrivalent vaccine have completed 5 years of follow-up [63]. At 5 years, the combined incidence of HPV 6-, 11-, 16-, and 18-related persistent infection or disease was reduced in vaccine-recipients by 96%, and no vaccine recipient developed HPV 6-, 11-, 16-, or 18-related precancerous cervical dysplasia or genital warts.

As the quadrivalent vaccine is the only one available at the time of this publication, the following recommendation can only be applied to it. The CDC's Advisory Committee on Immunization Practices has recommended routine vaccination of females aged 11 to 12 years with three doses of quadrivalent HPV vaccine, but it can be started in girls as young as 9 years of age [60]. The three vaccination series is given at 0, 2, and 6 months. It is preferable that the vaccine be administered before sexual activity or known exposure to HPV for optimal benefit. "Catch-up" vaccination is recommended for women aged 13 to 26 years who have not been previously vaccinated or who have not completed the three vaccine series. Vaccination provides less protection to those who have already been infected with one or more of the four vaccine HPV types. However, vaccination is still recommended, as these will still be protected against the other vaccine subtypes. In opposition to the CDC's guidelines, the American Cancer Society does not recommend universal vaccination among women aged 19 to 26 years, because of a probable reduction in efficacy as the number of lifetime sexual partners rise [64].

References

[1] Aral SO, Holmes K, Padian NF, et al. Overview: individual and population approaches to the epidemiology and prevention of sexual transmitted diseases and human immunodeficiency virus infection. J Infect Dis 1996;174(2):127–33.

[2] Center for Disease Control and Prevention. Sexually transmitted disease surveillance 2005. Atlanta, GA: US Department of Health and Human Services, CDC; 2006. Available at: http://www.cdc.gov/nchstp/dstd/stats_trends/stats_and_trends.htm. Accessed October 31, 2007.

[3] Weinstock H, Berman S, Cates W Jr. Sexually transmitted diseases among American youth: incidence and prevalence estimates, 2000. Perspect Sex Reprod Health 2004;36(1):6–10.

[4] Centers for Disease Control and Prevention, Workowski KA, Berman SM. Sexually transmitted diseases treatment guidelines, 2006. MMWR Recomm Rep 2006;55(RR-11):1–94.

[5] Mawhorter SD. Travel medicine for the primary care physician. Cleve Clin J Med 1997;64(9):483–92.

[6] Berg E, Benson DM, Haraszkiewicz P, et al. High prevalence of sexually transmitted diseases in women with urinary infections. Acad Emerg Med 1996;3(11):1030–4.

[7] Marrazzo JM, Koutsky LA, Stine KL, et al. Genito human papilloma virus infection in women who have sex with women. J Infect Dis 1998;178(6):1604–9.

[8] Perez G, Skurnick JH, Denny TN, et al. Herpes simplex type II and mycoplasma genitalium as risk factors for heterosexual HIV transmission: report from the heterosexual HIV transmission study. Int J Infect Dis 1998;3(1):5–11.

[9] Centers for Disease Control and Prevention. Expedited partner therapy in the management of sexually

transmitted diseases. Atlanta (GA): US Department of Health and Human Services; 2006.

[10] DiCarlo RP, Martin DH. The clinical diagnosis of genital ulcer disease in men. Clin Infect Dis 1997; 25(2):292–8.

[11] Langenberg AG, Corey L, Ashley RI, et al. A prospective study of new infections with herpes simplex virus type 1 and type 2. Chiron HSV Vaccine Study Group. N Engl J Med 1999;341:1432–8.

[12] White C, Wardropper AG. Genital herpes simplex infection in women. Clin Dermatol 1997;15(1): 81–91.

[13] Baker DA. Diagnosis and treatment of viral STD's in women. Int J Fertil 1997;42(2):107–14.

[14] Margesson LJ. Vulvar disease pearls. Dermatol Clin 2006;24(2):144–55.

[15] Benedetti J, Corey L, Ashley R. Recurrence rates in genital herpes after symptomatic first-episode infection. Ann Intern Med 1994;121:847–54.

[16] Wald A, Ashley-Morrow R. Serological testing for herpes simplex virus (HSV)-1 and HSV-2 infection. Clin Infect Dis 2002;35(Suppl 2):S173–82.

[17] Morrow RA, Friedrich D, Krantz E, et al. Development and use of a type-specific antibody avidity test based on herpes simplex virus type 2 glycoprotein G. Sex Transm Dis 2004;31(8):508–15.

[18] Schmid GP. Treatment of chancroid. Clin Infect Dis 1999;28(Suppl 1):S14–20.

[19] Hart G. Syphilis tests in diagnostic and therapeutic decision making. Ann Intern Med 1986;104:368–76.

[20] Golden M, Marra C, Holmes K. Update on syphilis: resurgence of an old problem. JAMA 2003;209(11): 1510–5.

[21] Hicks CB, Benson PM, Lupton GP, et al. Seronegative secondary syphilis in a patient infected with the human immunodeficiency virus with Kaposi Sarcoma: a diagnostic dilemma. Ann Intern Med 1987;107:492–5.

[22] Erbelding EJ, Vlahov D, Nelson KE, et al. Syphilis serology in human immunodeficiency virus infection: evidence for false negative fluorescent treponemal testing. J Infect Dis 1997;176(5):1397–400.

[23] Calonge N. Screening for syphilis infection: recommendation statement. U.S. Preventive Services Task Force. Ann Fam Med 2004;2:362–5.

[24] Greenblatt RM, Lukehart SA, Plummer FA, et al. Genital ulceration as a risk factor for human immunodeficiency virus infection. AIDS 1988;2(1): 47–50.

[25] Stamm WE, Handsfield HH, Rompalo AM, et al. The association between genital ulcer disease and acquisition of HIV infection in homosexual men. JAMA 1988;260(10):1429–33.

[26] Mabey D, Peeling RW. Lypmhogranuloma venerum. Sex Transm Infect 2002;357:1831–6.

[27] Berger RE, Alexander ER, Harnisch JP, et al. Etiology, manifestations and therapy of acute epididymitis: prospective study of 50 cases. J Urol 1979;121: 750–4.

[28] Rees E. Treatment of pelvic inflammatory disease. Am J Obstet Gynecol 1980;138:1042–7.

[29] Simms I, Stephenson JM. Pelvic inflammatory disease epidemiology: what do we know and what do we need to know? Sex Transm Infect 2000;76:80–7.

[30] Scholes D, Stergachis A, Heidrich FE, et al. Prevention of pelvic inflammatory disease by screening for cervical chlamydial infection. N Engl J Med 1996; 334:1362–6.

[31] Johnson RE, Newhall WJ, Papp JR, et al. Screening tests to detect Chlamydia trachomatis and Neisseria gonorrhoeae infections. MMWR Recomm Rep 2002;51(RR-15):1–38.

[32] Van der Pol B, Martin DH, Schachter J, et al. Enhancing the specificity of the COBAS AMPLICOR CT/NG test for *Neisseria gonorrhoeae* by retesting specimens with equivocal results. J Clin Microbiol 2001;39:3092–8.

[33] Centers for Disease Control and Prevention. Increases in fluoroquinolone-resistant Neisseria gonorrhoeae— Hawaii and California, 2001. MMWR Morb Mortal Wkly Rep 2002;51:1041–4.

[34] Centers for Disease Control and Prevention. Update to CDC's sexually transmitted diseases treatment guidelines, 2006: fluoroquinolones no longer recommended for treatment of gonococcal infections. MMWR Morb Mortal Wkly Rep 2007;56(14): 332–6.

[35] World Health Organization. Global incidence and prevalence of selected curable sexually transmitted infections: overview and estimates. Geneva (IL): WHO; 2001.

[36] Cotch MF, Pastorek JG 2nd, Nugent RP, et al. Trichomonas vaginalis associated with low birth weight and preterm delivery. The Vaginal Infections and Prematurity Study Group. Sex Transm Dis 1997; 24(6):353–60.

[37] Sorvillo F, Kerndt P. Trichomonas vaginalis and amplification of HIV-1 transmission. Lancet 1998; 351(9097):213–4.

[38] Potts JM, Ward AM, Rackley RR. Association of chronic urinary symptoms in women and ureaplasma urealyticum. Urology 1999;55(4):486–9.

[39] Taylor-Robinson D, Furr PM. Update on sexually transmitted mycoplasmas. Lancet 1998;351(3):12–5.

[40] Colli E, Landoni M, Parazzini F. Treatment of male partners and recurrence of bacterial vaginosis: a randomised trial. Genitourin Med 1997;3(4): 267–70.

[41] Hanson JM, McGregor JA, Hillier SL, et al. Metronidazole for bacterial vaginosis. A comparison of vaginal gel vs. oral therapy. J Reprod Med 2000; 45(11):889–96.

[42] Ho GYF, Bierman R, Beardsley L, et al. Natural history of cervicovaginal papilloma virus infection in young women. N Engl J Med 1998;338:423–8.

[43] Frydenberg M, Malek RS. Human papilloma virus infection and its relationship to carcinoma of the penis. Urologe A 1993;7:185–98.

[44] Syrjanen KJ, Heinonen UM, Kauraniemi T. Cyto-logic evidence of the association of condylomatous lesions with dysplastic and neoplastic changes in the uterine cervix. Acta Cytol 1981;25:17–22.

[45] Adam E, Berkova ZD, Axnerova Z, et al. Papilloma-virus detection: demographic and behavioral charac-teristics influencing the identification of cervical disease. Am J Obstet Gynecol 2000;182:257–64.

[46] Kulasingham SL, Hughes JP, Kiviat NB, et al. Eval-uation of human papillomavirus testing in primary screening for cervical abnormalities: comparison of sensitivity, specificity, and frequency of referral. JAMA 2002;288:1749–57.

[47] Walboomers JM, Jacobs MV, Manos MM, et al. Human papilloma virus is a necessary cause of inva-sive cervical cancer worldwide. J Pathol 1999;189: 12–9.

[48] Frisch M, Glimelius B, van deen Brule AJ, et al. Sexually transmitted infection as a cause of anal cancer. N Engl J Med 1997;337(19):1350–8.

[49] Schneider A, Kirchmayr R, DeVilliers EM, et al. Subclinical human papillomavirus infection in male sexual partners of female carriers. J Urol 1988;140:1431–4.

[50] Campion MJ, Singer A, Clarkson PK, et al. Increased risk of cervical neoplasia in consorts of men with penile condylomata acuminata. Lancet 1985;1:943–6.

[51] Arican O, Suneri F, Bilgie K, et al. Topical imiquimod 5% cream in external genital warts: a randomized, double-blind, placebo-controlled study. J Dermatol 2004;31(8):627–31.

[52] Langley PC, Tyring SK, Smith MH. The cost effective-ness of patient applied versus provider administered intervention strategies for the treatment of external genital warts. Am J Manag Care 1999;5:69–77.

[53] Perry CM, Lab HM. Topical imiquod: a review of its use in genital warts. Drugs 1999;58:375–90.

[54] Wiley DJ, Doughlas J, Beutner K, et al. External genital warts: diagnosis, treatment and prevention. Clin Infect Dis 2002;35:S210–24.

[55] Cardamakis E, Kotoulas IG, Metalinos K, et al. Treatment of urethral condylamata acuminate or flat condylomata with interferon. J Urol 1994;152:2011–3.

[56] Metawea B, El-Nashar AR, Kamel I, et al. Applica-tion of viable Bacille Calmette-Guerin topically as a potential therapeutic modality in condylomata acuminate: a placebo controlled study. Urology 2005;65(20):247–50.

[57] Markowitz LE, Dunne EF, Saraiya M, et al. Quadri-valent human papillomavirus vaccine: recommenda-tions of the Advisory Committee on Immunization Practices (ACIP). MMWR Recomm Rep 2007; 56(RR-2):1–24.

[58] Joura EA, Leodolter S, Hernandez-Avila M, et al. Efficacy of a quadrivalent prophylactic human papil-lomavirus (types 6, 11, 16, and 18) L1 virus-like-particle vaccine against high-grade vulval and vaginal lesions: a combined analysis of three rando-mised clinical trials. Lancet 2007;369(9574):1693–702.

[59] Garland SM, Hernandez-Avila M, Wheeler CM, et al. Quadrivalent vaccine against human papillo-mavirus to prevent anogenital diseases. N Engl J Med 2007;356:1928–43.

[60] The FUTURE II Study Group. Quadrivalent vac-cine against human papillomavirus to prevent high-grade cervical lesions. N Engl J Med 2007; 356:1915–27.

[61] Villa LL, Costa RLR, Petta CA, et al. Prophylactic quadrivalent human papillomavirus (types 6, 11, 16, and 18) L1 virus-like particle vaccine in young women: a randomised double-blind placebo-con-trolled multicentre phase II efficacy trial. Lancet Oncol 2005;6(5):271–8.

[62] Harper DM, Franco EL, Wheeler CM, et al. Sustained efficacy up to 4.5 years of a bivalent L1 virus-like particle vaccine against human papilloma-virus types 16 and 18: follow-up from a randomised control trial. Lancet 2006;367:1247–55.

[63] Villa LL, Costa RLR, Petta CA, et al. High sus-tained efficacy of a prophylactic quadrivalent human papillomavirus types 6/11/16/18 L1 virus-like parti-cle vaccine through 5 years of follow-up. Br J Cancer 2006;95(11):1459–66.

[64] Saslow D, Castle PE, Cox JT, et al. American Can-cer Society guideline for human papillomavirus (HPV) vaccine use to prevent cervical cancer and its precursors. CA Cancer J Clin 2007;57:7–28.

ELSEVIER
SAUNDERS

Urol Clin N Am 35 (2008) 47–58

UROLOGIC
CLINICS
of North America

New Developments in the Diagnosis and Management of Pediatric UTIs

Ross Bauer, MD*, Barry A. Kogan, MD

*Division of Urology, Department of Urology, Albany Medical College, 23 Hackett Boulevard,
Albany, NY 12208–3499, USA*

Urinary tract infections (UTIs) in children are common and a major source of morbidity. The incidence of UTIs in childhood is not precisely known because it is not a reportable disease, and in many cases, especially in infants, UTIs are probably underdiagnosed. Furthermore, the definitions and criteria for diagnosis vary considerably; for example, should children with asymptomatic bacteriuria be included, or what criteria should be used to diagnose a UTI when the urine is obtained with a bagged urine specimen [1]. Nonetheless, it has been estimated that 7% of girls and 2% of boys have a UTI prior to age 6 [2]. During the first year of life more boys than girls are diagnosed with a UTI, with uncircumcised boys having a 10-fold greater risk than those circumcised [2]. This trend reverses after the first year of life, with more girls than boys being diagnosed with a UTI.

Pediatric UTIs constitute a significant health burden, although the actual costs are not known [3]. In the United States, overall inpatient hospital costs are estimated to be greater than $180 million alone. This fails to include the costs of follow-up, including imaging, or the costs to society of parents losing productivity for diagnosis, treatment, and follow-up of their child's infection [3–5].

This article reviews the diagnosis and work-up of UTIs in children, and presents current data reviewing the roles of radiologic imaging, surgical correction, and antibiotic prophylaxis in the setting of pediatric UTIs.

Diagnosis of urinary tract infections in children

Early and rapid diagnosis is paramount to initiating prompt antimicrobial therapy and thereby limiting renal damage. In children, however, the diagnosis is in no way straightforward. UTIs are found in more than 5% of infants and young children who have no source of fever from history or physical examination [6], and in another study of febrile infants, 13.6% were found to have infections of the urine. The symptoms of a UTI in young children, however, are very nonspecific. Rarely are symptoms referable to the urinary tract observed. Even in older children UTIs rarely present with dysuria (more likely a sign of introital irritation) or urgency. Instead, frequency and urgency may be manifest as new-onset or increased incontinence. Likely, many UTIs are either not diagnosed or diagnosed late. Because the symptoms can be quite obscure, it is important that primary care providers have a high index of suspicion for UTIs in children [6].

It is well recognized that a well-collected urinary specimen is critical to make the diagnosis of infection; however, a noncontaminated specimen is hard to obtain in children. There are four ways that urine may be obtained: (1) a bagged specimen, where a bag is taped to the perineum and urine obtained after the child voids (obviously useful in infants, but there is a high risk of obtaining a contaminated sample); (2) a midstream collection (unreliable in children, especially young girls and uncircumcised boys in whom contaminated samples are likely) is useful if negative, but if positive, it is hard to tell whether the collection was contaminated; (3) a catheterized specimen (obviously traumatic in children and

* Corresponding author.
E-mail address: bauerr@mail.amc.edu (R. Bauer).

0094-0143/08/$ - see front matter © 2008 Elsevier Inc. All rights reserved.
doi:10.1016/j.ucl.2007.09.007

urologic.theclinics.com

further, in the uncooperative girl it can easily be contaminated); and (4) suprapubic aspiration (clearly the least likely to be contaminated, but again, traumatic in children and rarely practiced in the current, litigious environment).

Four determinants from the urinalysis have been accepted as supporting a UTI: (1) positive urinary leukocyte esterase on dipstick (revealing the presence of white blood cells in the urine), which has a sensitivity and specificity of about 75% [7]; (2) positive urinary nitrite on dipstick (dietary nitrates are reduced to nitrite by many gram-negative urinary bacteria), the sensitivity is low at 60% although the specificity approaches 100% [7]; (3) more than five white blood cells per high-powered field on microscopic examination of the spun urinary sediment; and (4) any bacteria seen on a high-powered examination of the spun urinary sediment. The presence of any bacteria on Gram stain has a sensitivity of 93% and specificity of 95%, better than dipstick evaluation for leukocyte esterase and nitrite [8]. Microscopic examination of the sediment can also reveal epithelial cells (strongly suggestive of contamination) or white blood cell casts (pathognomonic of pyelonephritis) [6].

The urine culture is a critical part of the workup for a presumed UTI. The culture identifies the organism causing the infection and helps guide treatment with the correct antibiotics. The traditional definition for a clinically significant UTI is more than 100,000 cfu/mL [6]. Lower numbers have also been shown to correlate with a UTI, especially when obtained by suprapubic aspirate. Lower numbers can also constitute a UTI because of additional factors (eg, hydrational dilution and frequent voiding) [6].

Distinguishing upper from lower tract urinary tract infections

Traditionally, clinical grounds have been used to distinguish pyelitis and pyelonephritis from cystitis. In particular, when urinary frequency and dysuria are accompanied by flank pain and a high-grade fever ($>38.5°C$) and rigors, this suggests the diagnosis of pyelonephritis [9]. These clinical findings are not entirely reliable, however, in identifying that the kidney is involved. Similarly, urinalysis, C-reactive protein, and erythrocyte sedimentation rate have low predictive value. More recently, there has been interest in identifying new markers to help identify acute pyelonephritis.

Cytokines are small proteins that help initiate the inflammatory process and have been identified as markers of infections and inflammation. The most recognized are tumor necrosis factor-α and interleukin-6 [10]. Although initially promising as markers of upper tract infection, they were ultimately shown to have low sensitivity and specificity for upper tract infections.

More promising is procalcitonin (PCT). PCT is a polypeptide identical to the prohormone of calcitonin that has been described as a potential marker for biologic disease [11,12]. PCT is a 116-amino acid propeptide of calcitonin that lacks hormonal activity. Plasma concentrations in healthy subjects, chronic inflammatory states, viral infections, and autoimmune disease are below 0.5 ng/mL. In moderate localized bacterial infection PCT ranges from 0.5 to 2, and in severe gram-negative bacterial infections with sepsis and multiorgan failure the level is found to be above 2 ng/mL [13].

Bacterial cells produce a cell wall, and all bacterial cell walls contain peptidoglycan. Gram-negative bacteria contain an extra layer in the cell wall structure called the outer membrane, which is outside the peptidoglycan layer. Endotoxin is a component of this outer membrane and is released in gram-negative infections. The most common organisms associated with UTI and pyelonephritis are the gram-negative bacteria *Escherichia coli*, *Proteus* sp, and *Pseudomonas* sp, which all produce endotoxin. Gram-positive organisms including *Staphylococcus aureus* and *Enterococcus faecalis* are also known to cause pyelonephritis but do not form or release endotoxin [6]. It has been shown that PCT is present in the serum 2 to 6 hours after the release of bacterial endotoxin into the bloodstream and its half-life in serum ranges from 24 to 30 hours [14]. The plasma concentration of PCT reaches a peak in 6 hours and stays high as long as the infectious stimulus is present. Because of its relatively short half-life, a rapid downfall is apparent by 48 hours after successful antibiotic treatment [13].

Correlations between PCT and pyelonephritis have now been well demonstrated. PCT levels have been found to be increased significantly in children with febrile UTI, and levels greater than 0.5 ng/mL were found when renal parenchyma involvement was present [15]. PCT has also been evaluated to distinguish risk of scarring in the setting of UTI. In those with UTI and no scarring, PCT levels remained low. In contrast, those with renal scarring had elevated initial PCT levels that remained elevated for at least 24 hours [16]. Further large multicenter studies are needed to validate the previous studies, determine its use in gram-positive infections, and better delineate sensitivity and specificity rates, but PCT is promising as a useful tool in differentiating pyelonephritis from cystitis in children.

Renal imaging

It has long been recognized that UTIs in the pediatric population may serve as a marker for anatomic abnormalities. Obstructive lesions are found in 5% to 10% of children with reflux and in 21% to 57% of children with UTIs [6]. Hence, imaging has been thought to be appropriate after the diagnosis of a UTI in a young child. There has been considerable controversy, however, over which children to image. A consensus published in the *Journal of Pediatrics* in 1999 provided practice parameters for infants and young children 2 months to 2 years of age with UTIs. These guidelines stated that infants and young children 2 months to 2 years of age with UTIs who do not demonstrate the expected clinical response within 2 days of antimicrobial therapy should undergo ultrasonography promptly, and either voiding cystourethrography (VCUG) or radionuclide cystography should be performed at the earliest convenient time, and young children 2 months to 2 years of age with UTIs who have the expected response to antimicrobials should have a sonogram and either VCUG or radionuclide cystography performed at the earliest convenient time [17].

Ultrasound

Ultrasonography can be used to identify many renal abnormalities, such as abnormalities of renal size and shape, duplication anomalies, hydronephrosis, or hydroureters. The bladder is also evaluable with ultrasound and may show thickening or the presence of other abnormalities like bladder diverticula or ureteroceles [17]. These findings may diagnose an abnormality or may suggest a problem like vesicoureteral reflux (VUR). Further, Doppler ultrasonography (and so-called power Doppler ultrasonography) can also be used to detect small areas of inflammation within the kidney, essentially diagnosing acute pyelonephritis. Unfortunately, the sensitivity and specificity of ultrasound for acute pyelonephritis is not very good [18]. An important caveat of renal-bladder ultrasound is that it is dependent on the skill of the operator, so it is important to have technicians and radiologists who have experience with both ultrasound and pediatric patients [6].

Even so, it has been argued that ultrasound may not be needed after UTIs in young children, perhaps because many have had prenatal ultrasounds that have demonstrated normal kidneys [19,20]. The authors' study of their population has confirmed that ultrasound remains a highly useful study. In their experience, it altered the diagnosis and treatment in at least 4.4% of patients [21]. Because it is noninvasive and radiation free, it is an excellent study in young children with UTIs.

Voiding cystourethrogram

Because VUR is seen in up to 50% of children with pyelonephritis, a VCUG has been thought to be a most important examination for children with clinical pyelonephritis. It has been shown that normal children have a very low rate of VUR ($<1\%$), whereas those with pyelonephritis have a much higher rate [22]. The test is considered invasive because it requires urethral catheterization. Because of this, parents and pediatricians have for many years questioned its necessity. Many techniques have been tested for reducing the trauma of the test, including hypnosis and sedation with midazolam [23,24]. Because these techniques greatly increase the time, cost, and risk of the test, they have not been widely adopted.

Radiation exposure has also been an issue. The test may be done with either traditional fluoroscopic techniques or with a radioisotope [6]. The radionuclide cystogram has traditionally had approximately 1/100th of the radiation exposure. Further, because imaging is continuous with a radionuclide cystogram (versus intermittent with fluoroscopy), it seems to be more sensitive in determining reflux than a traditional contrast VCUG [25,26]. Fluoroscopic VCUG is more accurate at grading reflux, however, and can show spinal abnormalities, bladder and urethral anatomy, periureteral diverticula, and other upper tract detail that cannot be identified with radionuclide cystography [6]. Traditionally, fluoroscopic VCUG has been the choice over radionuclide cystography in boys where urethral abnormalities may be present and for the initial study in girls [17]. More recently, new fluoroscopic equipment and tailored techniques have reduced the difference in radiation exposure and have led to more widespread adoption of the traditional VCUG [27,28]. Ultrasonographic techniques, including using microbubbles as a contrast agent, have been attempted, but have not been found to be useful [29]. Similarly, techniques that avoid catheterization, including ultrasound and indirect radionuclide methodologies, have not been found to be useful [30]. In the authors' experience, the traditional fluoroscopic VCUG remains an important study for children with febrile UTIs.

Tc 99m dimercaptosuccinic acid renal scanning

A positive urine culture is the gold standard for identifying a UTI. Determining whether the infection affects the kidneys, however, has been difficult. Radionuclide scanning using Tc 99m dimercaptosuccinic (DMSA) has become readily available and is used in many centers to help diagnose acute pyelonephritis [31].

Renal scintigraphy using DMSA has been shown to be accurate in detecting acute pyelonephritis and renal scarring in both animal models of acute pyelonephritis and in humans [32,33]. DMSA when injected intravenously binds to renal proximal tubular cells, and when radiolabeled, renal cortical images can be obtained 2 to 4 hours later. An area of decreased uptake in the kidney represents an area of abnormal or damaged renal tubular cells. These radionuclide scans have been compared with histopathology specimens, have an overall sensitivity and specificity of 86% and 91% for diagnosing acute pyelonephritis in animal studies, and have theoretical benefits over other types of studies for this purpose [34,35].

Scans may be used in the acute setting to determine the degree and site of involvement of a UTI. Many initial DMSA defects, however, resolve on follow-up. DMSA scans also may be used to determine the presence and extent of permanent damage (scarring) after an episode of pyelonephritis by imaging several months after the infection. DMSA scans have been shown to be several times more sensitive in the detection of renal scarring than the intravenous pyelogram or ultrasound [36]. Although the study is associated with relatively high doses of radiation to the kidneys, the radiation exposure to the ovaries and bone marrow is minimal [37]. CT has been proposed as an alternative, but is thought to have higher radiation exposure overall [38].

Although clearly the best study for determining the presence of renal scarring, the role of DMSA scanning has come into question. In an era of cost-benefit analysis, the question is whether the results of the study alter management.

In most cases the answer is no, hence the study may not be needed. The presence of scarring, however, may be an indication that reflux is more likely to persist and the study may be beneficial for this purpose. A study supporting the use of DMSA scanning revealed abnormal scans in 42% of patients with first-time UTIs and in 55% of patients with recurrent UTIs [39]. Three categories of abnormalities were noted: (1) renal cortical defects, (2) dilated pelvicalyceal system, and (3) renal swelling showing disproportionate function compared with size. The study concluded that the high yield of renal abnormalities by Tc 99m DMSA scanning emphasizes the importance of scanning all cases of UTIs, including patients with a first-time infection. The authors concluded that the pattern of abnormalities in the scan may help in planning for subsequent management of UTIs in these patients [39].

In further support of DMSA scanning, Nguyen and coworkers [40] compared renal ultrasound results with DMSA results in 34 patients with known sterile reflux. The study found most infants with high-grade reflux had decreased differential function or cortical defects on DMSA. Parenchymal defects detected by Tc 99m DMSA renal scintigraphy were often not identified by renal ultrasound. The study concluded that Tc 99m DMSA renal scintigraphy is especially useful for initially evaluating infants with high-grade, sterile VUR. Further, several studies have demonstrated that renal status, as documented by radionuclide scanning, is predictive of reflux resolution, with normal kidneys being associated with a higher rate of reflux resolution [41,42].

In Wales, a DMSA scan is a mandatory part of the work-up for a UTI in those children less than 7 years of age. A study out of Wales, however, questioned the validity of DMSA scanning in children greater than 1 year old because only 2% of those children were found to have renal scarring. Their final conclusion was that only those children with signs of pyelonephritis should undergo a DMSA scan [43].

Recommendations for imaging

At this time, guidelines at Albany Medical Center for imaging in the pediatric community following UTI are as follows:

Routine tailored VCUG for
  • Children younger than 5 years of age with a febrile UTI

- Males of any age with a first UTI
- Girls younger than the age of 2 years with a first UTI
- Children with recurrent UTI

Renal ultrasonography for
- Children younger than 5 years old with a febrile UTI
- Males of any age with a first UTI
- Girls younger than the age of 3 years with a first UTI
- Children with recurrent UTI
- Children with a UTI who do not respond promptly to therapy to determine whether a renal abscess or obstruction is present

Routine DMSA scanning
- DMSA scanning is warranted in selected cases in which the diagnosis of UTI is uncertain on account of equivocal urinalysis or culture results (eg, in patients receiving antimicrobial therapy at the time the urine culture is obtained) and in newborns with reflux
- Follow-up scintigraphy to establish the presence of scarring is not routinely necessary, because the significance and management of scarring seen only on a DMSA scan has not been studied adequately; however, in high-risk populations, such as infants with febrile UTIs or those children with high-grade reflux, this study may well have prognostic significance

New and somewhat experimental approaches to imaging

There are some new ideas, primarily as regards the use of VCUGs. There is an effort to avoid or at least limit their use. One approach is to use DMSA scanning and ultrasound acutely. If the DMSA scan shows a renal injury, a VCUG is needed. If the DMSA is negative, even acutely after a clinical episode of pyelonephritis, it suggests that scarring in the future is unlikely [44,45]. Hence, some argue that a VCUG is unnecessary. In theory, if the principal reason for diagnosing and treating reflux is to prevent scarring, then there is no need to diagnose or treat reflux in those cases. If there is a normal DMSA scan, no VCUG is necessary in those cases. Some argue that these patients, even if they do not get scarring, likely will have recurrent pyelonephritis and it is worthwhile to diagnose reflux in these patients, if only

to put them on prophylactic antibiotics for a period of time (see later).

Another approach is to increase the time between VCUGs in children with known reflux. Traditionally, studies have been performed annually to evaluate for resolution of reflux. It has been proposed that every 2 years is a more reasonable approach and this limits both catheterization and radiation exposure in the child [46].

Finally, there is limited information on what to expect in a child who has had a complete radiographic work-up that is negative. The authors found that about 20% of these children will have recurrent UTIs despite negative radiologic evaluation. Although not statistically significant, there is a trend for an increased recurrence risk in girls and particularly those with a history of recurrent febrile illnesses [47]. The significance of these recurrent infections has not been determined.

Treatment of reflux

VUR is a common problem, yet its importance and treatment remain confusing after many years of study. The relevance of reflux deals with the question of recurrent pyelonephritis and potentially renal scarring as a result. One of the big challenges faced is the decision to treat or not to treat a particular child. Traditional therapy included long-term prophylactic antibiotic treatment to prevent infections along with observation, in anticipation of the child outgrowing the reflux. As more was learned about voiding and bowel dysfunction, treatment of "elimination dysfunction" was emphasized in addition to traditional therapy. High spontaneous resolution rates can be obtained, especially for lower grades of reflux, but admittedly with the cost of long-term use of antimicrobials and repeated imaging with VCUGs. Surgical indications were "breakthrough" UTIs or failure of resolution of reflux over years. Surgery was associated with considerable morbidity and some complications, hence in a randomized trial, the International Study of Reflux in Children, there were few differences between the groups. The principal findings were that the rate of scarring and infections was similar in both groups, but the rate of clinical pyelonephritis was lower in the surgical group. The rate of surgical complications was much higher in Europe than in the United States [48]. A recent meta-analysis showed similar results. Ten trials were identified involving 964 children. These trials compared long-term antibiotics and surgical correction of VUR with antibiotics (seven trials); antibiotics with no treatment (one trial); and different materials for endoscopic correction of VUR (two trials). Risk of UTI by 1 to 2 and 5 years was not significantly different between surgical and medical groups. Surgical treatment did result in a 60% reduction in febrile UTI by 5 years but no concomitant significant reduction in risk of new or progressive renal damage at 5 years.

In 1997 the American Urological Association convened the Pediatric Vesicoureteral Reflux Guidelines Panel to make a set of guidelines to determine when to treat reflux medically versus surgically [49]. Table 1 reviews the guidelines for treatment with no renal scarring present, and Table 2 presents the recommendations when renal scarring is present.

As seen from the recommendations, surgery is recommended for higher grades of reflux. Different surgical treatment options are available to these patients. The standard surgical care has always been open surgical repair (eg, ureteral reimplantation). In the past, the problems with open surgical procedures for reflux were that they required many days of catheterization, required many days of hospitalization, and were associated with severe dysuria postoperatively. Attempts have been made to minimize the morbidity and the extravesical approach has been proposed. The extravesical detrussorhapy is highly successful and reduces the morbidity greatly, but there is a 3% to 4% rate of retention when done for bilateral reflux [50,51]. It is usually reserved for cases of unilateral reflux. Nonetheless, with modern surgical and anesthetic techniques open transvesical reimplantation can be done with 23-hour stays or even as an outpatient [52]. Success rates for either technique are about 98% for curing reflux. These developments, combined with a general tendency to avoid over use of antibiotics, have resulted in a trend toward earlier surgery. This has been accentuated even more by the use of laparoscopic techniques in some centers [53,54].

This trend, although promising, has come into question with the advent of endoscopic treatment of reflux. The STING procedure was introduced years ago and has been used successfully in Europe using polytef paste as a bulking agent [55]. The procedure requires anesthesia, but is minimally invasive, takes only minutes, and has a high rate of curing reflux, particularly because a second and even third injection can be done

easily in the case of initial failure. Because of scattered reports of possible complications related to the polytef, that substance has never been approved for use in the United States. After an extensive search for alternative agents, dextranomer/hyaluronic acid (Dx/HA) copolymer was approved by the US Food and Drug Administration in 2001 for use for this purpose [56].

This agent consists of dextranomer microspheres of an average size of 80 to 250 μm in sodium hyaluronic acid solution. Each milliliter of mixture consists of 0.5 mL microspheres and 0.5 mL sodium hyaluronan. This substance is biodegradable, has no immunogenic properties, and seems to have no potential to cause malignant transformation. Results vary with some reporting success rates of 90% for individual ureters, but most studies showing success rates of around 70% for curing reflux. Long-term reflux resolution rates are not known because it is difficult to restudy patients who are doing well, but there does seem to be a small recurrence rate after 1 year [57].

Whether endoscopic Dx/HA copolymer treatment should supplant open surgery remains controversial. The success rate of open surgery is still significantly higher and for many open surgeries, postoperative VCUGs are not needed in routine cases. With success rates of 70% to 90% reported, however, VCUGs remain essential for endoscopic treatment. In some parents' perception, the need for VCUG diminishes the benefits of the endoscopic treatment. At this time, in the authors' practice this decision is a family driven choice.

The advent of endoscopic, minimally invasive treatment, however, may have further shifted reflux care in general. If 70% to 90% of patients can be cured with a low-risk, 15-minute procedure with minimal morbidity, one must question whether it is appropriate to continue patients on the traditional management of long-term antimicrobials and repeated testing over years. Although not accepted broadly, there has been a subtle shift in the paradigm of treatment and early endoscopic treatment may be considered appropriate soon.

Not all VUR needs intervention and treatment does not always prevent complications [58]. In one small study no significant differences in risk for UTI or renal damage were found between antibiotic prophylaxis and no treatment [59]. For now, patients continue to be treated according to the guidelines shown in Tables 1 and 2 [49], but the role of intervention continues to be evaluated and new guidelines are currently under development.

Table 1
Guidelines for treatment with no renal scarring present

Clinical Presentation		Treatment — Initial (antibiotic prophylaxis or open surgical repair)			Follow-up (continued antibiotic prophylaxis, cystography, or open surgical repair[a])		
Reflux Grade/laterality	Pt. age (y)	Guideline	Preferred option	Reasonable alternative	Guideline[b]	Preferred option[b]	No consensus[c]
I-II/Unilat. or bilat.	Younger than 1	Antibiotic prophylaxis					Boys and girls
	1-5	Antibiotic prophylaxis					Boys and girls
	6-10	Antibiotic prophylaxis					Boys and girls
III-IV/Unilat. or bilat.	Younger than 1	Antibiotic prophylaxis			Bilat.: surgery if persistent		
	1-5	Unilat.: antibiotic prophylaxis	Bilat.: antibiotic prophylaxis			Unilat.: surgery if persistent Surgery if persistent	
	6-10		Unilat.: antibiotic prophylaxis Bilat.: surgery	Bilat.: antibiotic prophylaxis		Surgery if persistent	
V/Unilat. or bilat.	Younger than 1		Antibiotic prophylaxis		Surgery if persistent		
	1-5		Bilat.: surgery Unilat.: antibiotic prophylaxis	Bilat.: antibiotic prophylaxis Unilat.: surgery	Surgery if persistent		
	6-10	Surgery					

[a] For patients with persistent uncomplicated reflux after extended treatment with continuous antibiotic therapy.

[b] See Duration of Reflux regarding the time that clinicians should wait before recommending surgery.

[c] No consensus was reached regarding the role of continued antibiotic prophylaxis, cystography, or surgery.

From Elder JS, Peters CA, Arant B Jr, et al. Pediatric vesicoureteral reflux guidelines panel summary report on the management of primary vesicoureteral reflux in children. J Urol 1997;157:1849; with permission.

Table 2
Recommendations when renal scarring is present

Clinical Presentation		Treatment					
		Initial (antibiotic prophylaxis or open surgical repair)			Follow-up (continued antibiotic prophylaxis, cystography, or open surgical repair[a])		
Reflux Grade/laterality	Pt. age (y)	Guideline[b]	Preferred option	Reasonable alternative	Guideline[b]	Preferred option[b]	No consensus[c]
I–II/Unilat. or bilat.	Younger than 1	Antibiotic prophylaxis					Boys and girls
	1–5	Antibiotic prophylaxis					Boys and girls
	6–10	Antibiotic prophylaxis					Boys and girls
III–IV/Unilat.	Younger than 1	Antibiotic prophylaxis			Girls: surgery if persistent	Boys: surgery if persistent	
	1–5	Antibiotic prophylaxis			Girls: surgery if persistent	Boys: surgery if persistent	
	6–10		Antibiotic prophylaxis		Surgery if persistent		
III–IV/Bilat.	Younger than 1	Antibiotic prophylaxis			Surgery if persistent		
	1–5		Antibiotic prophylaxis	Surgery	Surgery if persistent		
	6–10	Surgery					
V/Unilat. or bilat.	Younger than 1		Antibiotic prophylaxis	Surgery	Surgery if persistent		
	1–5	Bilat.: surgery	Unilat.: surgery			Surgery if persistent	
	6–10	Surgery					

[a] For patients with persistent uncomplicated reflux after extended treatment with continuous antibiotic therapy.

[b] See Duration of Reflux regarding the time that clinicians should wait before recommending surgery.

[c] No consensus was reached regarding the role of continued antibiotic prophylaxis, cystography, or surgery.

From Elder JS, Peters CA, Arant B Jr, et al. Pediatric vesicoureteral reflux guidelines panel summary report on the management of primary vesicoureteral reflux in children. J Urol 1997;157:1850; with permission.

Antibiotic prophylaxis

VUR is a very common problem in the pediatric urologic practice, and is usually initially managed with antibiotic prophylaxis with the anticipation of either spontaneous or surgical resolution. Surgical intervention has normally been reserved for those children who have febrile breakthrough UTIs, progression of renal scarring, noncompliance with medical therapy, or nonresolution of VUR after prolonged follow-up. All children with VUR have classically been placed on antibiotic prophylaxis until resolution. There is a group of children with continued reflux who remain clinically stable, have normal elimination habits, and VUR is of low to mid grade. These children may be at low risk of UTI and reflux may not impact on renal outcome. In addition, there exists parental pressure to justify the continued use of antibiotic prophylaxis in stable children with VUR [60].

In a nonrandomized review of 196 patients with VUR treated with and without prophylactic antibiotics, the infection rate on and off of antibiotics was 0.29 and 0.24 UTIs per patient per year, respectively [61]. Similar results were seen out of Canada in 2005 [60] and Children's Hospital of Philadelphia in 1999 [62]. The pediatric urologic community has started to question the need for antibiotic prophylaxis in this population, with the caveat that the long-term outcome of children with persistent reflux off antibiotics remains unknown, especially for females who may well enter their sexually active and reproductive years with reflux. Studies now are investigating the role of antibiotic prophylaxis, even in higher-risk populations. In one multicenter, randomized controlled study, 236 patients aged 3 months to 18 years with acute pyelonephritis were randomly assigned to receive urinary antibiotic prophylaxis or not. Although the study has some flaws, no statistically significant differences were found among the groups with respect to rate of recurrent UTI, type of recurrence, rate of subsequent pyelonephritis, and development of renal parenchymal scars over 1 year of follow-up [22]. With the continued growth of multidrug-resistant bacteria, the role of antibiotic prophylaxis will continue to be questioned and researched in the coming years and as noted, at least one study has questioned the need for antimicrobials, even in very young children [22].

Circumcision

The role of circumcision continues to be debated among physicians and the public. The most recent statement by the American Academy of Pediatrics is as follows: "Circumcision is not essential to a child's well-being at birth, even though it does have some potential medical benefits. These benefits are not compelling enough to warrant the AAP to recommend routine newborn circumcision. Instead, we encourage parents to discuss the benefits and risks of circumcision with their pediatrician, and then make an informed decision about what is in the best interest of their child" [63]. Proponents of circumcision believe in it for religious beliefs, infection reduction, cosmetic effects, and prevention of penile cancer. In contrast, opponents state that it is not beneficial medically and places the patient, most often an infant, under unnecessary pain and suffering [6]. In 1999 in the United States, 65.3% of all male newborns born in hospitals were circumcised [64]. For most of the past 20 years, proportionately more white newborns received circumcisions than did black infants, but this has gradually equalized so that by 1999, the latest year data are available, 65.5% of white newborns and 64.4% of black newborns were circumcised [64]. Newborn circumcision rates continue to vary greatly by geographic region. In the past 20 years, 81% of babies born in the Midwest underwent circumcisions. In contrast, in the West only 37% had a circumcision [64].

In relation to circumcision and UTIs, it is well accepted that circumcision reduces the rate of UTI in the first 6 months by about 10-fold [65–67]. The etiology of this benefit is a little unclear. It has been shown that there is bacterial colonization of the foreskin during the first 6 months of life that may be an important risk factor for the development of UTIs. Colonization decreases after the first 6 months of life, probably because the foreskin often becomes retractable around that age. Further, uropathogens are known to adhere to and readily colonize the mucosal surface of the foreskin but not the keratinized shaft skin [63].

The question of whether circumcision helps to prevent infections later in life also continues to be debated throughout the literature. The most recent data in 2005 reviewed over 400,000 children identified from 12 studies and found that circumcision does reduce the risk of UTI [68]. The degree of risk reduction that is present varies, however, based on the patient. Normal boys have a risk of infection of about 1%, meaning 111 boys need to be circumcised to prevent one UTI. Boys known to have either recurrent UTI or high-grade VUR have a risk of UTI recurrence of 10% and 30% and the numbers-needed-to-treat are 11 and 4, respectively. Circumcision is not without complications, however, and hemorrhage and infection are most common, occurring at rate of about 2%. Taking into account the benefits and dangers of circumcision, net clinical benefit was found to be likely only in boys at high risk of UTI [68].

The role of circumcision in the prevention of HIV has been described in multiple studies in adult men. Most recently studies from Africa have reported lower rates of HIV infection in those who are circumcised. Three randomized studies of circumcision in young men all had to be stopped early because of an approximately 60% risk reduction in the rate of HIV infection [69]. All these studies were done in adult men in high-risk populations. How well they translate to neonates in the United States is unclear. Consideration of this should be given to future studies of neonates.

At this time, the recommendation for circumcision for boys is as follows:

- Multiple documented UTIs with no other source noted
- Neonates with a documented high risk for pyelonephritis, including those with genitourinary abnormalities and high-grade reflux
- Children who may be at high risk for HIV infection

Summary

UTIs in children are common and cause significant morbidity. They are challenging to diagnose and a high index of suspicion is required. Prompt antimicrobial therapy is uniformly accepted for renal and other symptomatic infections, but the type of imaging to be performed has been getting more controversial over time. Finally, therapy for VUR has undergone considerable modification with some recommending very early endoscopic treatment and others recommending observation without prophylactic antibiotics. Ongoing clinical trials will help decipher the future direction in this area.

References

[1] Siegel N. Rudolph's pediatrics. In: Rudolph C, editor. Kidney and urinary tract. New York: McGraw-Hill; 2003.

[2] Marild S, Jodal U. Incidence rate of first-time symptomatic urinary tract infection in children under 6 years of age. Acta Paediatr 1998;87:549–52.

[3] Hellerstein S. Acute urinary tract infection: evaluation and treatment. Curr Opin Pediatr 2006;18: 134–8.

[4] Freedman AL. Urologic Diseases in North America Project: trends in resource utilization for urinary tract infections in children. J Urol 2005;173: 949–54.

[5] Freedman AL. Urinary tract infection in children. In: Litwin SC, editor. Urological diseases in America. Washington, DC: US Department of Health And Human Service, Public Health Service, National Institute of Health, National Institute of Diabetes and Digestive Kidney Diseases; 2007. p. 441.

[6] Linda S. Urinary tract infections in infants and children. In: Walsh P, editor. 8th edition. Campbell's urology, vol. 3. Baltimore (MD): Saunders; 2002. p. 1846–84.

[7] Downs SM. Technical report: urinary tract infections in febrile infants and young children. The Urinary Tract Subcommittee of the American Academy of Pediatrics Committee on Quality Improvement. Pediatrics 1999;103:e54.

[8] Gorelick MH, Shaw KN. Screening tests for urinary tract infection in children: a meta-analysis. Pediatrics 1999;104:e54.

[9] Stunell H, Buckley O, Feeney J, et al. Imaging of acute pyelonephritis in the adult. Eur Radiol 2007; 17:1820–8.

[10] Gurgoze M, Akarsu S, Yilmaz E, et al. Proinflammatory cytokines and procalcitonin in children with acute pyelonephritis. Pediatr Nephrol 2005; 1445–8.

[11] Assicot M, Gendrel D, Carsin H, et al. High serum procalcitonin concentration in patients with sepsis and infection. Lancet 1993;515–8.

[12] Karsai W, Oberhölffer M, Meier-Hellman A, et al. Procalcitonin: a new indicator of systemic response to severe infections. Infection 1997;329–34.

[13] Pecile P, Romanello C. Procalcitonin and pyelonephritis in children. Curr Opin Infect Dis 2007;20: 83–7.

[14] Dandona P, Nix D, Wilson MF, et al. Procalcitonin increase after endotoxin injection in normal subjects. J Clin Endocrinol Metab 1994;79:1065–8.

[15] Benador N, Siegrist CA, Gendrel D, et al. Procalcitonin is a marker of severity of renal lesions in pyelonephritis. Pediatrics 1998;102:1422–5.

[16] Prat C, Dominguez J, Rodrigo C, et al. Elevated serum procalcitonin values correlate with renal scarring in children with urinary tract infection. Pediatr Infect Dis J 2003;22:438–42.

[17] Committee on Quality Improvement S. o. U.T.I. Practice parameter: the diagnosis, treatment, and evaluation of the initial urinary tract infection in febrile infants and young children. Pediatrics 1999; 103:843–52.

[18] Dolezel Z, Mach V, Kopecna L, et al. [Diagnosis of acute pyelonephritis in childhood: comparison of ultrasonographic examination and renal scintigraphy using 99mTc DMSA]. Bratisl Lek Listy 2000; 101:495–8 [in Czech].

[19] Hoberman A, Charron M, Hickey RW, et al. Imaging studies after a first febrile urinary tract infection in young children. N Engl J Med 2003;348: 195–202.

[20] Alon US, Ganapathy S. Should renal ultrasonography be done routinely in children with first urinary tract infection? Clin Pediatr (Phila) 1999;38:21–5.

[21] Giorgi LJ Jr, Bratslavsky G, Kogan BA. Febrile urinary tract infections in infants: renal ultrasound remains necessary. J Urol 2005;173:568–70.

[22] Garin EH, Olavarria F, Garcia Nieto V, et al. Clinical significance of primary vesicoureteral reflux and urinary antibiotic prophylaxis after acute pyelonephritis: a multicenter, randomized, controlled study. Pediatrics 2006;117:626–32.

[23] Butler LD, Symons BK, Henderson SL, et al. Hypnosis reduces distress and duration of an invasive medical procedure for children. Pediatrics 2005; 115:e77–85.

[24] Stokland E, Andreasson S, Jacobsson B, et al. Sedation with midazolam for voiding cystourethrography in children: a randomised double-blind study. Pediatr Radiol 2003;33:247–9.

[25] McLaren CJ, Simpson ET. Direct comparison of radiology and nuclear medicine cystograms in young infants with vesico-ureteric reflux. BJU Int 2001;87: 93–7.

[26] Unver T, Alpay H, Biyikli NK, et al. Comparison of direct radionuclide cystography and voiding cystourethrography in detecting vesicoureteral reflux. Pediatr Int 2006;48:287–91.

[27] Lederman HM, Khademian ZP, Felice M, et al. Dose reduction fluoroscopy in pediatrics. Pediatr Radiol 2002;32:844–8.

[28] Ward VL. Patient dose reduction during voiding cystourethrography. Pediatr Radiol 2006;36:168–72.

[29] Correas JM, Claudon M, Tranquart F, et al. The kidney: imaging with microbubble contrast agents. Ultrasound Q 2006;22:168–72.

[30] Sixt R, Stokland E. Assessment of infective urinary tract disorders. Q J Nucl Med 1998;42:119–25.

[31] Nammalwar BR, V M, Sankar J, et al. Evaluation of the use of DMSA in culture positive UTI and culture negative acute pyelonephritis. Indian Pediatr 2005; 42:691–6.

[32] Craig JC, Wheeler DM, Irwig L, et al. How accurate is dimercaptosuccinic acid scintigraphy for the diagnosis of acute pyelonephritis? A meta-analysis of experimental studies. J Nucl Med 2000;41:986–93.

[33] Kogan BA, Kay R, Wasnick RJ, et al. 99m Tc-DMSA scanning to diagnose pyelonephritic scarring in children. Urology 1983;21:641–4.

[34] Ditchfield M, Summerville D, Grimwood K, et al. Time course of transient cortical scintigraphic

defects associated with acute pyelonephritis. Pediatr Radiol 2002;32:849–52.

[35] Stoller ML, Kogan BA. Sensitivity of 99m technetium-dimercaptosuccinic acid for the diagnosis of chronic pyelonephritis: clinical and theoretical considerations. J Urol 1986;135:977–80.

[36] Shaikh N, H A. Clinical features and diagnosis of urinary tract infections in children. In: UpToDate, 2007.

[37] Arnold RW, Subramamian G, McAfee JG, et al. Comparison of Tc99m complexes for renal imaging. J Nucl Med 1975;16:357–67.

[38] Majd M, Nussbaum Blask AR, Markle BM, et al. Acute pyelonephritis: comparison of diagnosis with 99mTc-DMSA, SPECT, spiral CT, MR imaging, and power Doppler US in an experimental pig model. Radiology 2001;218:101–8.

[39] Loutfi I, Al-Zaabi K, Elgazzar AH. Tc-99m DMSA renal scan in first-time versus recurrent urinary tract infection-yield and patterns of abnormalities. Clin Nucl Med 1999;24:931–5.

[40] Nguyen HT, Bauer SB, Peters CA, et al. 99m Technetium dimercapto-succinic acid renal scintigraphy abnormalities in infants with sterile high grade vesicoureteral reflux. J Urol 2000;164:1678–9.

[41] Godley ML, Desai D, Yeung CK, et al. The relationship between early renal status, and the resolution of vesico-ureteric reflux and bladder function at 16 months. BJU Int 2001;87:457–62.

[42] Yeung CK, Sreedhar B, Sihoe JD, et al. Renal and bladder functional status at diagnosis as predictive factors for the outcome of primary vesicoureteral reflux in children. J Urol 2006;176:1152–6.

[43] Deshpande PV, Jones KV. An audit of RCP guidelines on DMSA scanning after urinary tract infection. Arch Dis Child 2001;84:324–7.

[44] Rushton HG. The evaluation of acute pyelonephritis and renal scarring with technetium 99m-dimercaptosuccinic acid renal scintigraphy: evolving concepts and future directions. Pediatr Nephrol 1997;11: 108–20.

[45] Godbole P, SG, Wagstaff J. Investigating febrile UTI's in infants: is a cystogram necessary. Abstracts of the ESPU XVIIIth Annual Congress, Brugge, Belgium; April 25–28, 2007.

[46] Thompson M, Simon SD, Sharma V, et al. Timing of follow-up voiding cystourethrogram in children with primary vesicoureteral reflux: development and application of a clinical algorithm. Pediatrics 2005; 115:426–34.

[47] Bratslavsky G, Feustel PJ, Aslan AR, et al. Recurrence risk in infants with urinary tract infections and a negative radiographic evaluation. J Urol 2004;172:1610–3, discussion 1613.

[48] Jodal U, Smellie J, Lax H, et al. Ten-year results of randomized treatment of children with severe vesicoureteral reflux. Final report of the International Reflux Study in Children. Pediatr Nephrol 2006;21: 785–92.

[49] Elder JS, Peters CA, Arant B Jr, et al. Pediatric ves-icoureteral reflux guidelines panel summary report on the management of primary vesicoureteral reflux in children. J Urol 1997;157:1846–51.

[50] Zaontz MR, Maizels M, Sugar EC, et al. Detrusor-rhaphy: extravesical ureteral advancement to correct vesicoureteral reflux in children. J Urol 1987;138:947–9.

[51] Fung LC, McLorie GA, Jain U, et al. Voiding effi-ciency after ureteral reimplantation: a comparison of extravesical and intravesical techniques. J Urol 1995;153:1972–5.

[52] Putman S, Wicher C, Wayment R, et al. Unilateral extravesical ureteral reimplantation in children per-formed on an outpatient basis. J Urol 2005;174:1987–9, discussion 1989–90.

[53] Yeung CK, Sihoe JD, Tam YH, et al. Laparoscopic excision of prostatic utricles in children. BJU Int 2001;87:505–8.

[54] Ng JW, Yeung CK, et al. Laparoscopic excision of pelvic kidney with single vaginal ectopic ureter. J Pediatr Surg 1998;33:1731–2.

[55] Puri P. Ten year experience with subureteric Teflon (polytetrafluoroethylene) injection (STING) in the treatment of vesico-ureteric reflux. Br J Urol 1995;75:126–31.

[56] Elder JS, Diaz M, Caldamone AA, et al. Endoscopic therapy for vesicoureteral reflux: a meta-analysis. I. Reflux resolution and urinary tract infection. J Urol 2006;175:716–22.

[57] Lackgren G, Wahlin N, Stenberg A. Endoscopic treatment of children with vesico-ureteric reflux. Acta Paediatr Suppl 1999;88:62–71.

[58] Lorenzo AJ, Khoury AE. Endoscopic treatment of reflux: management pros and cons. Curr Opin Urol 2006;16:299–304.

[59] Wheeler DM, VD, Hodson EM, et al. Interventions for primary vesicoureteric reflux. In: Cochrane Database Syst Rev 2004.

[60] Al-Sayyad AJ, Pike JG, Leonard MP. Can prophy-lactic antibiotics safely be discontinued in children with vesicoureteral reflux? J Urol 2005;174:1587–9, discussion 1589.

[61] Thompson RH, Chen JJ, Pugach J, et al. Cessa-tion of prophylactic antibiotics for managing per-sistent vesicoureteral reflux. J Urol 2001;166:1465–9.

[62] Cooper CS, Chung BI, Kirsch AJ, et al. The out-come of stopping prophylactic antibiotics in older children with vesicoureteral reflux. J Urol 2000;163:269–72, discussion 272–3.

[63] Shapiro E. American academy of pediatrics policy statements on circumcision and urinary tract infec-tion. Rev Urol 1999;1:154–6.

[64] Trends in circumcisions among newborns. Edited by U.S.D.O.H.A.H. SERVICES Centers for Disease Control and Prevention, 2007. Available at: www.cdc.gov.nchs/products/pubs/pubd/hestatak/cicumcisions/circumcisions.htm.

[65] Schoen EJ, Colby CJ, Ray GT. Newborn circumci-sion decreases incidence and costs of urinary tract in-fections during the first year of life. Pediatrics 2000;105:789–93.

[66] Wiswell TE, Enzenauer RW, Holton ME, et al. De-clining frequency of circumcision: implications for changes in the absolute incidence and male to female sex ratio of urinary tract infections in early infancy. Pediatrics 1987;79:338–42.

[67] Roberts JA. Does circumcision prevent urinary tract infection. J Urol 1986;135:991–2.

[68] Singh-Grewal D, Macdessi J, Craig J. Circumci-sion for the prevention of urinary tract infection in boys: a systematic review of randomised trials and observational studies. Arch Dis Child 2005;90:853–8.

[69] Newell ML, Barnighausen T. Male circumcision to cut HIV risk in the general population. Lancet 2007;369:617–9.

ELSEVIER
SAUNDERS

Urol Clin N Am 35 (2008) 59–68

UROLOGIC
CLINICS
of North America

HIV-AIDS – Urologic Considerations

Steve Lebovitch, MD, Jack H. Mydlo, MD*

*Department of Urology, Temple University Hospital, 3401 North Broad St., Suite 330, Zone C,
Philadelphia, PA 19140, USA*

Since the early 1980s and the identification of HIV and AIDS, doctors and health care workers have struggled to treat this disease and its comorbidities. The virus has infected an estimated 39.5 million individuals worldwide, with an estimated 1.2 million people in the United States [1]. Since 1996 and the advent of combination therapy of antiretroviral medications, known as highly active antiretroviral therapy (HAART), patients who would have at one time died of renal failure caused by HIV nephropathy or opportunistic infections with atypical organisms are currently actively treated for quality-of-life conditions, such as voiding dysfunction, fertility, and erectile dysfunction (ED). The patient population living with HIV survives longer and experiences and needs treatment for expected age-related conditions. They have complications of the disease and the therapies they receive. Nephrolithiasis, a known complication of the protease inhibitors, has increased urologists involvement in caring for patients who have ureteral obstruction. Common age-related malignancies affect patients who have HIV, and as the population of HIV-positive patients lives longer, urologists may be asked about other malignancies, such as HIV-related lymphomas, which can cause ureteral obstruction, and Kaposi's sarcoma (KS), which involves the genitalia. This article reviews the urologist's involvement in the medical complications that have arisen from HIV or its treatment.

Urinary tract infections

Patients who have HIV experience a greater risk of urinary tract infections (UTIs) when their CD4 counts fall below 500/mm^3 [2,3]. Voiding dysfunction with urinary stasis is also implicated as a factor in the increased incidence of UTIs in HIV-positive patients [4]. A 17% incidence rate of UTI is seen in HIV-positive patients [4,5]. Patients may have bacteruria and be asymptomatic; however, common symptoms include dysuria, frequency, fever, and hematuria [3–6]. Patients with asymptomatic bacteria may not require treatment [6,7]. Common bacterial pathogens in HIV-infected patients are *Escherichia coli*, *Enterobacter* (Enterococci), *Pseudomonas aeruginosa*, *Proteus* spp, *Klebsiella*, *Acinetobacter*, *Staphylococcus aureus*, group D *Streptococcus*, *Serratia*, and *Salmonella* spp [3–7].

Disseminated infections may affect potentially any portion of the urinary tract. They are usually caused by atypical organisms and frequently associated with a depressed immune system. Atypical pathogens may include fungi (*Candida albicans*, *Aspergillus*, *Blastomyces*, *Cryptococcus neoformans*, *Cryptosporidia*, *Histoplasma capsulatum*), parasites (*Toxoplasma gondii*, *Pneumocystis carinii*), mycobacteria (*Mycobacterium tuberculosis*, *Mycobacterium avium* complex), and viruses (cytomegalovirus and adenovirus) [6–10]. Patients with urinary symptoms and negative urine culture results should be evaluated further with atypical culture and stain analysis. Treatment with culture-sensitive antibiotics is recommended when available.

Epididymitis, orchitis, and necrotizing fasciitis

Many HIV-positive patients present with inquiries about urethral infections related to sexually transmitted diseases, such as *Chlamydia trachomatis* and *Neisseria gonorrhoeae*. These infections can propagate and spread to cause epididymitis-orchitis. Other opportunistic and systemic

---

* Corresponding author.
E-mail address: jmydlo@temple.edu (J.H. Mydlo).

infections lead to abscess formation in the penoscrotal region. Organisms associated with suppurative and antibiotic resistant infections in this
population include cytomegalovirus, *Candida*,
mycobacterium, *Toxoplasmosis*, and *Salmonella*.
These infections, especially *Salmonella*, may be
difficult to eradicate and require lifelong suppressive therapy. Initial treatment recommendations
include a 2- to 4-week regimen of doxycycline,
100 mg, twice daily and ciprofloxacin, 500 mg,
twice daily [3].

Depending on the severity of the infection and
how immunocompromised an individual is, necrotizing fasciitis of the genitalia or Fournier's
gangrene may develop [11]. This aggressive infection may be the initial presentation of a patient
who has HIV. Immediate diagnosis with wide surgical débridement to healthy and viable tissue is
necessary. Broad-coverage antibiotics are used
until the organism and its sensitivities are obtained. Patients may require aggressive hemodynamic support, and multiple surgical
débridements may be necessary. A diverting colos-
tomy and eventual skin grafts may be necessary
for appropriate healing to take place.

Prostatitis

The algorithms used to treat basic urologic
conditions, such as prostatitis and chronic pelvic
pain syndrome, in HIV-positive patients are
similar to those used to treat non–HIV-positive
patients. In treating HIV-positive patients, however, evaluation and treatment of atypical organisms frequently are warranted. The incidence of
acute bacterial prostatitis is 1% to 2% in the
general population, whereas it is 3% in asymptomatic, HIV-infected patients and 14% in patients who have AIDS [4,12]. These data predate
treatment with HAART and likely are currently
lower in incidence. Patients who have acute prostatitis may experience fevers, dysuria, frequency,
malaise, urinary retention, and perineal pain
[3,4,12]. Digital rectal examination may indicate
an enlarged, tender, and potentially fluctuant
prostate [3,4,6,12]. In patients who have HIV,
the risk of developing a prostatic abscess or urosepsis is greater than in the general population because of the atypical pathogens previously
mentioned. They require increased monitoring
and evaluation and likely an extended duration
of culture-specific antimicrobial and antifungal
therapy [4,12]. If surgical intervention to drain
a prostatic abscess is necessary, it can be

accomplished by either transrectal or perineal aspiration or transurethral resection. Symptomatic
and disseminated fungal infections may require
long-term antifungal-directed therapy and prostatectomy [13]. As with all infections in immunocompromised patients, atypical pathogens
always should be considered.

Urolithiasis

Patients on HAART therapy are managed
with protease inhibitors, which act by preventing
terminal maturation in the formation of new viral
particles and are implicated as a cause of urolithiasis [14]. Indinavir, a protease inhibitor that has
been well investigated, is known to cause urolithiasis in 5% to 25% of HIV-positive patients
[14,15]. Metabolized mainly by the liver, 20% of
indinavir is not metabolized and is excreted in
the urine within 24 hours [4,16–19]. Indinavir
crystallizes when the pH of urine is more than 5
and the concentration is sufficient. Indinavir, as
a stone component, is seen only in 29% of calculi.
The remaining stone components are calcium oxalate, ammonium acid urate, and uric acid [20].
Although uncommon, pure indinavir calculi are
radiolucent on radiographic studies and there
may be minimal findings on noncontrast CT
studies [21].

Patients who have HIV also have metabolic
imbalances that may result in calculi formation.
Disturbances from malnutrition and diarrhea play
a role in dehydration, increase in urinary concentration, acidification, and hypocitraturia [20]. In
this metabolic state, stone formation is promoted.
Patients may present with flank pain and microscopic hematuria, which requires intravenous uro-
gram, renal ultrasonography, or a noncontrast
spiral CT scan. Renal collecting system dilation
may be the only radiologic finding in patients
with indinavir calculi, whereas other components
are seen as calcifications [4,6]. Conservative measures with hydration and analgesia may be effective in up to 80% of patients [19].

Once diagnosed with calculi, patients should
undergo a complete metabolic evaluation. Recommendations include not only stone analysis but also
two 24-hour urine collections for volume, calcium,
oxalate, uric acid, magnesium, phosphorous, and
sodium. Serum studies should be examined for
blood urea nitrogen, creatinine, calcium, and
serum electrolytes [20]. Recently, investigators
looked at the early plasma trough levels of indinavir in patients receiving 800 mg of indinavir three

times daily as a first-line protease inhibitor. Higher trough levels were associated with a higher rate of severe nephrolithiasis and a higher rate of all serious adverse reactions. Recommendations based on these conclusions included early indinavir trough determination and dose adjustment [22]. Stopping indinavir did not result in complete resolution of calculi formation or complications associated with them; therefore, patients rarely need treatment with an alternative drug [23].

When conservative management does not lead to resolution of symptoms or if a patient becomes acutely ill because of intractable pain, UTI, or high-grade obstruction, temporary stenting or nephrostomy tube placement is necessary. Manipulation with endoscopic stent placement may be enough to allow passage of these soft and gelatinous matrix stones, as in the case of pure indinavir stones [4]. Occasional ureteroscopic or percutaneous nephrolithotomy may be necessary for stone extraction.

Sexual dysfunction

ED and hypogonadism are recognized conditions in men who have HIV. Testicular atrophy is common and leads to infertility, ED, and decreased libido [6]. In one study that examined serum testosterone and ED in 300 such patients, 17% of men were hypogonadal. Increasing age and body mass index were positively associated with hypogonadism. The authors found no association between ED or hypogonadism and HIV therapy [24].

Testosterone supplementation has been used in testicular and hypothalamopituitary diseases for several decades. There has been growing interest in the use of testosterone in male contraception, aging, muscle-wasting conditions such as HIV, and ED [25]. The new transdermal patches, gels, and sustained-release buccal tablets are designed to provide testosterone levels that are close to normal physiologic levels [25]. These treatments, in addition to phosphodiesterase type-5 (PDE-5) inhibitors, can effectively treat men who have HIV and suffer from low libido caused by low levels of testosterone and ED.

Effective treatment of ED actually can be a factor in spreading the HIV virus. In one study by Karlovsky and colleagues [26], data obtained from the Centers for Disease Control and Prevention (CDC) in Atlanta demonstrated an increased incidence of gonorrhea among elderly men living in south Florida. Gonorrhea is a vehicle of transmission for HIV. Although there was not a direct correlation between the use of PDE-5 inhibitors and the increasing incidence of HIV among elderly men in south Florida, the association was suggested. Possible reasons may be that these elderly men grew up in the age before universal precautions and currently engage in risky behavior. Another example, in a study by Benotsch and colleagues [27], which discussed 304 homosexual men who engaged in sexual activity while on vacation or business trips, concluded that men who were taking PDE-5 medications reported higher rates of sexually risky behaviors.

HAART also plays a role in sexual dysfunction. Lamba and colleagues [28] found the incidence of ED and decreased libido in HIV-positive homosexual men to be 26%. In that study, in patients who were taking HAART, the incidence of reduced libido was 48% (caused by raised estradiol levels) and the rate of ED was 25%. Studies support and oppose the occurrence of sexual dysfunction in HIV-positive men taking HAART [29–31]. PDE-5 inhibitors also may have an interaction with indinavir and other protease inhibitors. In a report by Murray and colleagues [32], indinavir was a potent inhibitor of the hepatic mechanism of sildenafil. They suggested that starting sildenafil at a lower dose would be more appropriate in patients taking indinavir.

Men who are HIV positive are more likely to experience depression [33,34]. Depression is associated with low libido and ED, and common antidepressant medications, such as selective serotonin reuptake inhibitors, also decrease libido and sexual performance [35,36]. Knowing the effects on libido and sexual dysfunction, a PDE-5 inhibitor may be necessary to alleviate the sexual symptoms without interfering with depression therapy. The prescribing of PDE-5 inhibitors may allow patients to regain sexual activity and confidence, which can improve depressive symptoms. Subsequently, treatment with a lower dose of selective serotonin reuptake inhibitors may be possible [37,38].

Another aspect in treating patients who are HIV positive is the cost of the PDE-5 inhibitors. Because some insurance companies may not cover the cost of these pharmacotherapies, the financial burden of antiretroviral medications and PDE-5 inhibitors may fall primarily on the patient. Patients may opt for surgery, because they know a penile prosthesis is paid for by insurance, whereas the medication may not be [39]. There also may be somewhat of an ethical dilemma in treating HIV-positive patients for ED with either pharmacotherapy or surgery if a male patient does not have a steady committed partner and engages in risky behavior with multiple partners. By treating the ED condition, the physician may feel that he or she is essentially giving the patient a "loaded gun." A confidential, supportive doctor-patient relationship helps to improve patients' quality of life while trying to help stop the spread of the virus [40].

Urologists and other health care professionals who treat ED in HIV-positive patients face a significant challenge in trying to restore normal sexual function. It requires knowledge of the HIV disease and potential drug interactions and learning strategies aimed at reducing the infection rate. This interaction sometimes goes beyond the doctor-patient relationship to include careful consideration of the rights of the partner and society as a whole [39].

Fertility

With improving life expectancy on HAART, patients present with questions pertaining to fertility and disease transmission. Some patients have abnormal semen parameters associated with atrophy of the testes. Atrophy may be related to hypothalamopituitary axis dysfunction, inflammation, infection, chronicity of the disease, or malnutrition [4,41–43]. HIV has its own cytotoxic affect on germinal tissue and Sertoli cells, which leads to testicular atrophy.

Attention and counseling must be given to patients who have HIV and are interested in becoming parents. Transmission rates for unprotected heterosexual intercourse range from 1:1000 per contact (male/female) to less than 1:1000 (female/male) [44]. Options to minimize risk for horizontal and vertical transmission to offspring should be explained. For men infected with the virus, a method described by Semprini and colleagues in 1992, which involves sperm washing followed by assisted reproductive techniques, has proved to be the safest method to date [45,46]. Tested sperm carry a 10% risk of harboring the virus, which implies that patients are still at risk; in Europe, however, more than 500 children have been born after sperm washing, with zero seroconversions [44]. Mother-to-child transmission—or vertical transmission—can be minimized to less than 2% if cesarean section is performed along with intrapartum infusion of antiviral medications [6].

Voiding dysfunction

Early data on voiding dysfunction in HIV-positive patients indicated that few patients experienced disturbances in voiding; cases that involved dysfunction were usually associated with UTIs [47]. Patients do present to the primary physician or urologist complaining of lower urinary symptoms, such as dysuria, hesitancy, and decreased stream. Some patients at time of seroconversion experience various neurologic findings, including acute urinary retention. With disease progression patients may experience worsening micturition impairments. Disturbances may be related to recurrent or chronic UTI, central nervous system disturbances (eg, HIV encephalitis, cerebral toxoplasmosis, and HIV-related dementia), or peripheral neurologic deficits [4,6,47–49]. Central and peripheral neurologic causes account for approximately 61% of voiding dysfunction seen in affected patients [49]. AIDS-related malignancies or infectious processes, such as herpes and cytomegalovirus, are a few causes of common lower motor deficits usually seen [4].

Urodynamics may be useful in identifying underlying dysfunction. Common urodynamic findings identified by Hermieu and colleagues [49] included hypo- and hyperreflexia, acontractile hypoactive bladder, and detrusor-sphincter dyssynergia. Bladder hypocontractility was seen in 35% to 45% of patients at time of urinary retention. Outlet obstruction caused by prostatic enlargement only accounted for 18% of cases in patients with urinary retention. Treatment options for patients with outflow obstruction or hypo- and hyperreflexia can include intermittent catheterization until a patient's neurologic deficits prevent this task, at which time a chronic catheter or suprapubic cystotomy should be used. Outlet obstruction also can be treated with endoscopic methods when clinically indicated. Bladder hyperreflexia may be treated with anticholinergic agents as first-line therapy. Early reports indicated that patients who experience these abnormalities had a poor prognosis, with mortality usually within a mean of 8 years [3,49].

HIV-associated nephropathy

Despite HAART, kidney disease and renal failure are the fourth leading causes of death in HIV-positive patients [50]. Renal failure may be caused by metabolic dysfunction and volume depletion from chronic diarrhea, nephrotoxic medications, infections, ureteral obstruction from malignancies, and intrinsic diseases such as HIV-associated nephropathy. HIV-associated nephropathy occurs more frequently in HIV-positive black patients, with a black-to-white ratio of 12:1. HIV-associated nephropathy has become the third leading cause of end-stage renal disease among black patients aged 20 to 64, after diabetes and hypertension [51]. Characteristics include nephrotic disease with proteinuria more than 3.5 g/d and edema and hypertension. Renal ultrasound evaluation occasionally indicates kidney enlargement, but usually they are within normal size and have increased echogenicity. Diagnosis is confirmed with biopsy. Histologic findings may include a collapsing variant of focal segmental glomerulosclerosis, proliferation of renal tubular and visceral epithelial cells (podocytes), tubular microcystic formation, edema, interstitial fibrosis, and infiltration of the interstitium with leukocytes [52]. Patients progress rapidly, with end-stage renal disease with dialysis requirement occurring within 10 months of diagnosis. Despite hemodialysis, the 1-year-mortality rate is 50%; on antiretroviral therapy it still reaches approximately 30% [50]. Treatment includes HAART therapy for persons not on HIV medications and angiotensin-converting enzyme inhibitors. Medications that depend on renal breakdown and excretion should be adjusted with worsening renal insufficiency and failure.

Malignancies

The cancer rates in patients who have HIV have declined in the HAART era, but despite treatment, patients are still at higher risk for malignancies. Many mechanisms proposed that support malignancy formation include decreased immune surveillance, a direct effect of viral proteins, cytokine dysregulation, or other immunologic or viral cofactors [53,54] Patients are living into their sixth and seventh decades of life and are at a greater risk of malignancies than noninfected patients. Renal cell carcinoma, for example, carries an 8.5-fold greater risk for infected patients compared with noninfected patients [4,6,55].

A study by Engels and colleagues [56] assessed the relationship between HIV serostatus and the likelihood of developing KS, non-Hodgkin's lymphoma (NHL), or cervical cancer over time. Using registry data from the AIDS Cancer Match Registry Study and other cancer registries, comparisons were made between three different periods. Years 1980 to 1989, 1990 to 1995, and 1996 to 2002 were compared. The results of this study clearly showed that the risk of developing KS and NHL declined substantially over time; however, individuals who have HIV still maintained a higher risk of developing KS and NHL compared with persons in the general population. A second study followed a total of 59,101 individuals from 1992 to 2002 using data from various surveillance groups, such HIV Outpatient Study, a prospective observational study in HIV-positive patients, and the Surveillance and End Results project, which was composed of the general population. The results were compared to assess the relative risk of developing malignancies in the HIV-positive population. Risk was greatest in malignancies such as KS, lymphomas (Hodgkin's and non-Hodgkin's), cervical, liver, and testicular cancer, and melanoma. Of note, the researchers noted a decreased risk in patients who had HIV in relation to prostate and breast cancer [57].

Kaposi's sarcoma

KS is the most common HIV-related malignancy. Originally, in its classic form the disease was found in elderly men of Mediterranean or African background. Later it was seen in patients who were immunocompromised, such as transplant patients and persons who had with HIV/AIDS. Up to 20% of patients infected with HIV not being treated with HAART are affected by KS. This number is down approximately 90% from the pre-HAART era [58]. The human herpesvirus type 8, also known as KS-associated herpesvirus, is responsible for the development of KS. KS is rarely fatal. It arises from lymphatic endothelial cells that form vascular channels and give rise to the characteristic bruise-like appearing lesions [59]. KS, which more commonly occurs in men, can present as an indolent process, with minimal physical findingss or as a disseminated aggressive disease. Lesions usually present as red, black, purple, or brown nodules, macules, or patches that are typically painless but also can be ulcerating and painful. KS can present as a systemic disease that affects internal organs, including the kidneys [60] and testes [61].

Genital lesions appear in approximately 20% of patients who have KS [62]. Painful lesions can present on the penoscrotal region and cause edema and pain. Urethral meatal lesions may cause outlet obstruction and urinary retention.

Temporizing these patients with suprapubic cystotomy may be necessary until definitive treatment takes place [63]. Rare presentations of penile necrosis and gangrene have been reported as a result of vasculitis or vascular obstruction seen with progression of KS [64].

KS is not curable and treatment is either local or systemic. Primary treatment for KS involves initiation of HAART if patients have not started such treatment. Local treatment for cosmetically disturbing or painful lesions includes cryosurgery, vinca alkaloids, intralesional bleomycin or intralesional interferons, soft x-ray radiation, electron beam therapy, cobalt radiation (fractionated), retinoids, 9-cis-retinoic acid, and alitretinoin [58]. Systemic treatment for disseminated or visceral disease uses chemotherapeutic agents. The gold standard combination therapy of adriamycin, bleomycin, and vincristine has been replaced in recent years with liposomal anthracyclines, such as daunorubicin and doxorubicin [58]. In a recent study, the response rate of pegylated liposomal doxorubicin with HAART was 76% versus 20% in the HAART-only treatment group of patients who had advanced KS [65]. Paclitaxel is also effective in treating advanced KS and has a partial remission rate of 60% [66].

Immunotherapy is used for systemic treatment of KS with interferons. The efficacy of interferon treatment depends on the cellular immune status of a patient. Remission rates of 45% to 70% are seen. Studies indicate that to achieve remission rates of more than 45%, at least 400 CD4+ T cells/μL are needed [58]. Systemic therapies carry a greater risk for worsening of immunosuppression and opportunistic infections.

Lymphoma

Like KS, NHL is an AIDS-defining malignancy. Ninety percent of HIV-associated NHLs are of B-cell origin [67]. They are usually aggressive and when treated they are prone to recur. The incidence has decreased in patients taking HAART [57]. Patients may have lymphadenopathy, fevers, night sweats, and weight loss. NHL of the testes may present bilaterally and is usually disseminated at the time of diagnosis. Orchiectomy and radiation in combination with systemic chemotherapeutic agents are treatment options. The incidence of relapse and rapid progression is high in immunocompromised men. Renal involvement of NHL in patients who have AIDS is 6% to 12%, and presentation may be bilateral [4,6].

Ureteral obstruction from retroperitoneal lymphadenopathy is often diagnosed while evaluating renal failure and may require ureteral stenting or percutaneous nephrostomy drainage [4]. Complete remission is seen in 50% to 75% of patients with systemic treatment [67]. With relapse, progression can be rapid.

Testicular tumors

The prevalence of testicular tumors in immunocompromised patients ranges from 20 to 57 times that of the general population [4,6,68]. Germ cell testicular tumors are the third most common AIDS-related malignancy. A study that compared HIV-positive patients with a control population suggested that the incidence of seminoma is increased in men who have HIV [69]. In this population, testicular tumors may present bilaterally, as in NHL, and be disseminated at presentation. The difficulties experienced by practitioners pertain to the treatment of these malignancies and potential worsening of immunosuppression. HIV-positive patients, initially considered to be poor candidates for radiation and chemotherapy, are currently believed to have equal morbidity and response as patients who do not have HIV [4,68]. Patients should undergo treatment based on tumor histology and stage. With this in mind, patients may experience early mortality from disease recurrence or progression secondary to their underlying disease.

Dermatologic malignancies of the genitalia

HIV and human papillomavirus are sexually transmitted diseases with similar risk factors for transmission. Human papillomavirus types 16 and 18 are considered high risk in anogenital malignancy formation of carcinoma in situ and squamous cell carcinoma [70]. Carcinoma in situ of the penis, also known as Bowen's disease and considered a premalignant lesion, appears as a bright red or pink scaly patch on the glans or shaft. It should be treated with cryotherapy, topical 5-fluorouracil, laser therapy, or surgical excision. Squamous cell carcinoma is usually more aggressive in HIV-positive patients and should be excised and staged. Regional lymphadenectomy, radiation, or systemic chemotherapies should be used in a manner similar to treatment used for individuals not infected with HIV [71].

Prostate cancer

With increasing life expectancy, prostate cancer is expected to become an increasingly important health problem for men infected with HIV. Few cases are reported in the literature [72,73], so a definitive link between HIV and prostate cancer is uncertain. Early published data predated HAART therapy and indicated an increased risk for prostate cancer in the HIV-positive male population [7]. HIV with prostate cancer carried a poor prognosis, which was believed to be secondary to a patient's severely depressed immune system and hypogonadal state, which made androgen deprivation an ineffective therapy option. Some clinicians advocate screening patients in their early forties because of the potential for prostate cancer presenting in a disseminated manner with nonspecific features [73,74]. Patients can present with impaired constitutional symptoms, fever, weight loss, fatigue, and exertional dyspnea, despite having a sustained CD4+ count, having a contained viremia, and never requiring antiretroviral therapy. These patients are at risk for advanced, complicated, and widely metastatic disease with extensive bone marrow invasion, which precedes the appearance of local signs and symptoms that commonly lead to death.

Recently, Vianna and colleagues [75] examined a cohort of 534 men aged 49 years and older who had risk factors for HIV. Their goal was to determine the rate of and factors associated with elevated prostate-specific antigen levels. Serum prostate-specific antigen level and HIV serology and T-cell subsets for individuals who were HIV seropositive were measured. Three hundred ten patients were found to be HIV positive. Their statistical analysis found that prostate-specific antigen levels increased with age but did not differ by HIV status. The study recommended that standard prostate-specific antigen evaluations can be made with HIV-positive patients without the need for adjustments. Screening should take place at age 50 unless there is a family history or the patient is African American. A patient's prostate-specific antigen, Gleason score, HIV status, and comorbidities should be evaluated to plan treatment. Patients who are asymptomatic should be offered all possible treatment options, including surgery, radiation, androgen deprivation, and observation. Some clinicians believe that laparoscopic or robot-assisted surgery should be performed when possible to minimize risk of surgeon exposure [76].

Health care worker issues: prophylaxis and prevention of exposure and transmission

With appropriate precautions, health care–related seroconversion should not be a major concern for urologists. Documented occupational-acquired HIV infections are low; 57 occupational HIV infections were documented by the CDC [77]. Percutaneous injuries with hollow needles or cut injuries and mucous membrane exposure with infected blood carries the greatest of risk of transmission. The risk for HIV transmission after a percutaneous exposure to HIV-infected blood has been estimated to be approximately 0.3% (95% confidence interval [CI] = 0.2%–0.5%); after a mucous membrane exposure, the rate is approximately 0.09% (95% CI = 0.006%–0.5%) [78]. Urine carries low HIV titers, and there are no documented cases of seroconversion caused by this type of exposure.

To maintain low rates of HIV occupational transmission, the CDC has published preventive strategies to minimize occupational risks. The emphasis that all blood and body fluids are potentially infectious is at the heart of "Universal Precautions." Precautionary methods include barriers (ie, gloves, gowns), hand washing of contaminated areas after contact, and careful handling and disposing of sharps after their use. Despite the low transmission risk from urine, the use of a camera system during endoscopic procedures should be practiced.

The CDC has set up recommendations for HIV postexposure prophylaxis. Basic exposure that warrants postexposure prophylaxis (ie, exposure to mucous membranes or skin or a superficial percutaneous injury from a source who did not have end-stage AIDS or acute HIV illness) requires treatment with a 4-week, two-drug regimen (ie, zidovudine plus lamivudine). For exposures with increased risk of transmission (ie, high viral load from a source with a deep penetrating exposure), a three-drug regimen may be recommended. There are several combinations for three-drug regimens, and they should include two reverse transcriptase inhibitors (eg, zidovudine plus lamivudine) and a protease inhibitor (eg, lopinavir and ritonavir) [78].

These occupational exposures should be considered urgent medical concerns, and early intervention is essential. Although no randomized, controlled trials have compared one-, two-, and three-drug regimens, the CDC believes that prophylaxis is effective in preventing seroconversion in persons who received treatment within the initial 24 hours of exposure. Common side effects include nausea, fatigue, headache, and diarrhea. More toxic side effects include neutropenia, lactic acidosis, pancreatitis, and liver failure [78]. A meta-analysis of two- versus three-drug regimens indicated that the latter had a statistically significant worse side effect profile and a slight decrease in compliance [79]. All cases are not equal, and each hospital's employee health department should be consulted on treatment necessity and options.

Summary

In the era of HAART and diligent follow-up, patients diagnosed with HIV have a life expectancy of more than 20 years [80]. We are becoming more involved in the care of patients who have HIV and are severely immunocompromised. Knowledge of the various HIV manifestations of genitourinary conditions and treatment options benefits clinicians and improves patient outcomes.

References

[1] UNAIDS/WHO. AIDS epidemic update: December 2006. http://data.unaids.org/pub/EpiReport/2006/2006_EpiUpdate_en.pdf. Accessed May 20, 2007.

[2] Hoepelman AI, van Buren M, van den Broek J, et al. Bacteriuria in men infected with HIV-1 is related to their immune status (CD4+ cell count). AIDS 1992;6:179–84.

[3] Lee LK, Dinneen MD, Ahmad S. The urologist and the patient infected with human immunodeficiency virus or with acquired immunodeficiency syndrome. BJU Int 2001;88:500–10.

[4] Hyun G, Lowe FC. AIDS and the urologist. Urol Clin North Am 2003;30:101–9.

[5] Miles BJ, Melser M, Farah R, et al. The urological manifestations of the acquired immunodeficiency syndrome. J Urol 1989;142:771–3.

[6] Heyns CF, Fisher M. The urological management of the patient with acquired immunodeficiency syndrome. BJU Int 2005;95:709–16.

[7] Kwan DJ, Lowe FC. Acquired immunodeficiency syndrome: a venereal disease. Urol Clin North Am 1992;19:13–24.

[8] Steele BW, Carson CC. Recognizing the urologic manifestations of HIV and AIDS. Contemp Urol 1997;9:39–53.

[9] Kaplan MS, Wechsler M, Benson MC. Urologic manifestations of AIDS. Urology 1987;30:441–3.

[10] O'Regan S, Russo P, Lapointe N, et al. AIDS and the urinary tract. J Acquir Immune Defic Syndr 1990;3:244–51.

[11] Corman JM, Moody JA, Aronson WJ. Fournier's gangrene in a modern surgical setting: improved survival with aggressive management. BJU Int 1999;84:85–8.

[12] Leport C, Rousseau F, Perronne C, et al. Bacterial prostatitis in patients infected with the human immunodeficiency virus. J Urol 1989;141:334–6.

[13] Wise GJ, Shteynshlyuger A. How to diagnose and treat fungal infections in chronic prostatitis. Curr Urol Rep 2006;7(4):320–8.

[14] Hoffmann C, Mulcahy F. ART 2006. In: Hoffmann C, Rockstroh JK, Kamps SB, editors. HIV medicine 2006. Paris, Cagliari, Wuppertal: Flying; 2006. p. 284–5. Available at: http://www.HIVMEDICINE.com. Accessed May 20, 2007.

[15] Meraviglia P, Angeli E, Del Sorbo F, et al. Risk factors for indinavir-related renal colic in HIV patients: predictive value of indinavir dose/body mass index. AIDS 2002;16:2089–93.

[16] Heylen R, Miller R. Adverse effects and drug interactions of medications commonly used in the treatment of adult HIV-positive patients: part 2. Genitourin Med 1997;73:5–11.

[17] Tashima KT, Horowitz JD, Rosen S. Indinavir nephropathy. N Engl J Med 1997;336:138–9.

[18] Bruce RG, Munch LC, Hoven AD, et al. Urolithiasis associated with the protease inhibitor indinavir. Urology 1997;50:513–8.

[19] Daudon M, Estepa L, Viard JP, et al. Urinary stones in HIV-1 positive patients treated with indinavir. Lancet 1997;349:1294–5.

[20] Nadler RB, Rubenstein JN, Eggener SE, et al. The etiology of urolithiasis in HIV-infected patients. J Urol 2003;169:475–7.

[21] Schwartz BF, Schenkman N, Armenakas NA, et al. Imaging characteristics of indinavir calculi. J Urol 1999;161:1085–7.

[22] Collin F, Chene G, Retout S, et al. Indinavir trough concentration as a determinant of early nephrolithiasis in HIV-1-infected adults. Ther Drug Monit 2007;29(2):164–70.

[23] Kopp JB, Miller KD, Mican JM, et al. Crystalluria and urinary tract abnormalities associated with indinavir. Ann Intern Med 1997;127:119–25.

[24] Crum-Cianflone NF, Bavaro M, Hale B, et al. Erectile dysfunction and hypogonadism among men with HIV. AIDS Patient Care STDS 2007;21(1):9–19.

[25] Srinivas-Shankar U, Wu FCW. Drug insight: testosterone preparations. Nat Clin Pract Urol 2006;3(12):653–65.

[26] Karlovsky M, Lebed B, Mydlo JH. Increasing incidence and importance of HIV/AIDS and gonorrhea among men aged > 50 in the US in the era of erectile dysfunction therapy. Scan J Urol Nephrol 2004;38:247–52.

[27] Benotsch EG, Seeley S, Mikytuck JJ, et al. Substance use, medications for sexual facilitation, and sexual risk behavior among traveling men who

have sex with men. Sex Transm Dis 2006;33(12):706–11.

[28] Lamba H, Goldmeier D, Mackie NE, et al. Antiretroviral therapy is associated with sexual dysfunction and with increased serum estradiol levels in men. Int J STD AIDS 2004;15(4):234–7.

[29] Lallemand F, Salhi Y, Linard F, et al. Sexual dysfunction in 156 ambulatory HIV-infected men receiving highly active antiretroviral therapy combinations with and without protease inhibitors. J Acquir Immune Defic Syndr 2002;30(2):187–90.

[30] Schrooten W, Colebunders R, Youle M, et al. Eurosupport Study Group. Sexual dysfunction associated with protease inhibitor containing highly active antiretroviral treatment. AIDS 2001;15(8):1019–23.

[31] Sollima S, Oslo M, Muscia F, et al. Protease inhibitors and erectile dysfunction. AIDS 2001;15(17):2331–3.

[32] Murray C, Barry MG, Ryan M, et al. Interaction of sildenafil and indinavir when co-administered to HIV-positive patients. AIDS 1999;13(15):F101–7.

[33] Crum NF, Furtek JK, Olson PE, et al. A review of hypogonadism and erectile dysfunction and HIV-infected men during the pre-and post HAART eras: diagnosis, pathogenesis, and management. AIDS Patient Care STDS 2005;19(10):655–71.

[34] Alciati A, Gallo L, Monforte A, et al. Major depression-related immunological changes and combination antiretroviral therapy in HIVB-seropositive patients. Hum Psychopharmacol 2007;22(1):33–40.

[35] Shiri R, Koskomaki J, Tammela TL, et al. Bidirectional relationship between depression and erectile dysfunction. J Urol 2007;177(2):669–73.

[36] Fava M, Nurnberg HG, Seidman SN, et al. Efficacy and safety of sildenafil in men with serotonergic antidepressant associated erectile dysfunction: results from a randomized, double blind placebo controlled trial. J Clin Psychiatry 2006;67(2):240–6.

[37] Boyarsky BK, Haque W, Rouleau MR, et al. Sexual functioning in depressed outpatients taking mirtazapine. Depress Anxiety 1999;9(4):175–9.

[38] Ende AR, Lo Re V, DiNubile MJ, et al. Erectile dysfunction in an urban HIV-positive population. AIDS Patient Care STDS 2006;20(2):75–8.

[39] Nurnberg HG, Duttagupta S. Economic analysis of sildenafil citrate (Viagra) add-on to treat erectile dysfunction associated with selective serotonin reuptake inhibitor use. Am J Ther 2004;11(1):9–12.

[40] Sadeghi-Nejad H, Watson R, Irwin R, et al. Lecture 5: erectile dysfunction in the HIV-positive male. A review of medical, legal and ethical considerations in the age of oral pharmacotherapy. Int J Impot Res 2000;12(Suppl 3):S49–53.

[41] Lcibovitch I, Goldwasscr B. The spcctrum of acquired immunodeficiency syndrome-associated testicular disorders. Urology 1994;44:818–24.

[42] Pudney J, Anderson D. Orchitis and human immunodeficiency virus type I infected cells in reproductive tissues from men with the acquired immune deficiency syndrome. Am J Pathol 1991;139:149–60.

[43] DePaepe ME, Waxman M. Testicular atrophy in AIDS: a study of 57 autopsy cases. Hum Pathol 1989;20:210–4.

[44] Sonnenberg-Schwan U, Gilling-Smith C, Weigel M. HIV and wish for parenthood. In: Hoffmann C, Rockstroh JK, Kamps SB, editors. HIV medicine 2006. Paris, Cagliari, Wuppertal: Flying; 2006. p. 667–78. Available at: http://www.HIVMEDICINE.com. Accessed May 20, 2007.

[45] Semprini AE, Levi-Setti P, Bozzo M, et al. Insemination of HIV-negative women with processed semen of HIV-positive partners. Lancet 1992;340:1317–9.

[46] Garrido N, Meseguer M, Bellver J, et al. Report of the results of a 2 year programme of sperm wash and ICSI treatment for human immunodeficiency virus and hepatitis C virus serodiscordant couples. Hum Reprod 2004;19:2581–6.

[47] Gyrtrup HJ, Kristiansen VB, Zachariae CO, et al. Voiding problems in patients with HIV infection and AIDS. Scand J Urol Nephrol 1995;29:295–8.

[48] Menendez V, Espuna M, Perez A, et al. Neurogenic bladder in patients with acquired immunodeficiency syndrome. Neurourol Urodyn 1995;14:253–7.

[49] Hermieu JF, Delma V, Boccon-Gibod L. Micturition disturbances and human immunodeficiency virus infection. J Urol 1996;156:157–9.

[50] Rieke A. HIV and renal function. In: Hoffmann C, Rockstroh JK, Kamps SB, editors. HIV medicine 2006. Paris, Cagliari, Wuppertal: Flying; 2006. p. 571–84. Available at: http://www.HIVMEDICINE.com. Accessed May 20, 2007.

[51] Krieger JN. Urologic implications of AIDS and HIV infection. In: Wein AJ, Kavoussi LR, Novick AC, et al, editors. Campbell-Walsh urology. 9th edition. Philadelphia: Elsevier; 2006. p. 386–404.

[52] Shah SN, He CJ, Klotman P. Update on HIV-associated nephropathy. Curr Opin Nephrol Hypertens 2006;15:450–5.

[53] Blattner WA. Human retroviruses: their role in cancer. Proc Assoc Am Physicians 1999;111:563–72.

[54] Bellan C, De Falco G, Lazzi S, et al. Pathologic aspects of AIDS malignancies. Oncogene 2003;22:6639–45.

[55] Adjiman S, Zerbib M, Flam T, et al. Genitourinary tumors and HIV1 infection. Eur Urol 1990;18:61–3.

[56] Engels EA, Pfeiffer RM, Goedert JJ, et al for the HIV/AIDS Cancer Match Study. Trends in cancer risk among people with AIDS in the United States: 1980–2002. AIDS 2006;20(12):1645–54.

[57] Patel B, Hanson D, Novak R, et al. Incidence of AIDS defining and non-AIDS defining malignancies among IIIV-infected persons [abstract 813]. Presented at the 13th Conference on Retroviruses and Opportunistic Infections. Denver, Colorado, February 5–8, 2006.

[58] Schoefer H, Sachs DL. Kaposi's sarcoma. In: Hoffmann C, Rockstroh JK, Kamps SB, editors.

HIV medicine 2006. Paris, Cagliari, Wuppertal: Flying; 2006. p. 481–9. Available at. http://www. HIVMEDICINE.com. Accessed May 20, 2007.

[59] Tappero JW, Conant MA, Wolfe SF, et al. Kaposi's sarcoma: epidemiology, pathogenesis, histology, clinical spectrum, staging criteria and therapy. J Am Acad Dermatol 1993;28:371–95.

[60] Pollok RCG, Francis N, Cliff S, et al. Kaposi's sarcoma in the kidney. Int J STD AIDS 1995;6: 289–90.

[61] Weil DA, Ruckle HC, Lui PD, et al. Kaposi's sarcoma of the testicle. AIDS Read 1999;9(7): 455–61.

[62] Lowe FC, Lattimer DG, Metroka CE. Kaposi's sarcoma of the penis in patients with acquired immunodeficiency syndrome. J Urol 1989;142:1475–7.

[63] Swierzewski SJ III, Wan J, Boffini A, et al. The management of meatal obstruction due to Kaposi's sarcoma of the glans penis. J Urol 1993;150:193–5.

[64] Klein LT, Lowe FC. Penile gangrene associated with extensive Kaposi's sarcoma in patients with the acquired immunodeficiency syndrome. Urology 1995; 46:425–8.

[65] Martin-Carbonero L, Barrios A, Saballs P, et al. Pegylated liposomal doxorubicin plus highly active antiretroviral therapy versus highly active antiretroviral therapy alone in HIV patients with Kaposi's sarcoma. AIDS 2004;18:1737–40.

[66] Tulpule A, Groopman J, Saville MW, et al. Multicenter trial of low-dose paclitaxel in patients with advanced AIDS-related Kaposi sarcoma. Cancer 2002; 95:147–54.

[67] Hoffmann C. Malignant lymphomas. In: Hoffmann C, Rockstroh JK, Kamps SB, editors. HIV medicine 2006. Paris, Cagliari, Wuppertal: Flying; 2006. p. 491–503. Available at: http://www.HIVMEDICINE. com. Accessed May 20, 2007.

[68] Leibovitch I, Baniel J, Rowland RG, et al. Malignant testicular neoplasms in immunosuppressed patients. J Urol 1996;155:1938–42.

[69] Goedert JJ, Purdue MP, McNeel TS, et al. Risk of germ cell tumors among men with HIV/acquired immunodeficiency syndrome. Cancer Epidemiol Biomarkers Prev 2007;16(6):1266–9.

[70] Hausen HZ, Villiers ED. Human papilloma viruses. Annu Rev Microbiol 1994;48:427–47.

[71] Nguyen P, Vin-Christian K, Ming ME, et al. Aggressive squamous cell carcinomas in persons infected with the human immunodeficiency virus. Arch Dermatol 2002;138(6):827–8.

[72] O'Connor JK, Nedzi LA, Zakris EL. Prostate adenocarcinoma and human immunodeficiency virus: report of three cases and review of the literature. Clin Genitourin Cancer 2006;5(1):85–8.

[73] Manfredi R, Fulgaro C, Sabbatani S, et al. Disseminated, lethal prostate cancer during human immunodeficiency virus infection presenting with non-specific features: open questions for urologists, oncologists, and infectious disease specialists. Cancer Detect Prev 2006;30(1):20–3 [Epub 2006].

[74] Quatan N, Nair S, Harrowes F, et al. Should HIV patients be considered a high risk group for the development of prostate cancer? Ann R Coll Surg Engl 2005;87(6):437–8.

[75] Vianna LE, Lo Y, Klein RS. Serum prostate-specific antigen levels in older men with or at risk of HIV infection. HIV Med 2006;7(7):471–6.

[76] Levinson A, Nagler EA, Lowe FC. Approach to management of clinically localized prostate cancer in patients with human immunodeficiency virus. Urology 2005;65(1):91–4.

[77] CDC. Preventing occupational HIV transmission to healthcare personnel. February 2002. http://www.cdc.gov/hiv/resources/factsheets/hcwprev.htm. Accessed May 20, 2007.

[78] Panlilio AL, Cardo DM, Grohskopf LA, et al. Centers for Disease Control and Prevention: updated US Public Health Service guidelines for the management of occupational exposures to HIV and recommendations for postexposure prophylaxis. MMWR 2005; http://www.cdc.gov/mmwr/preview/mmwrhtml/rr5409a1.htm. Accessed May 20, 2007.

[79] Young T, Arens F, Kennedy G, et al. Antiretroviral post-exposure prophylaxis (PEP) for occupational HIV exposure. Cochrane Database Syst Rev 2007; 1:CD002835.

[80] Schackman BR, Gebo KA, Walensky RP, et al. The lifetime cost of current human immunodeficiency virus care in the United States [review]. Med Care 2006;44(11):990–7.

ELSEVIER
SAUNDERS

Urol Clin N Am 35 (2008) 69–79

UROLOGIC
CLINICS
of North America

Antibiotics in Urology – New Essentials

F.M.E. Wagenlehner, MD, PhD[a],*, W. Weidner, MD, PhD[a],
K.G. Naber, MD, PhD[b]

[a]Clinic of Urology and Pediatric Urology, Justus-Liebig-University, Rudolf-Buchheim-Str. 7,
35385 Giessen, Germany
[b]Technical University of Munich, Karl-Bickleder-Str. 44c, 94315 Straubing, Germany

Urinary tract infections (UTIs) are one of the most common reasons that adults seek medical and urologic consultation and are one of the most frequently occurring nosocomial infections [1–4]. In urology, nosocomial UTIs are almost exclusively complicated UTIs (ie, UTIs associated with structural or functional abnormalities of the urinary tract, with a broad spectrum of etiologic pathogens) [5]. Empirical antimicrobial therapy in urology must be instigated on occasions when urosepsis is pending or the general condition is deteriorated and is likely to improve significantly by the immediate use of antimicrobial agents [6]. For rational empiric therapy it is necessary to consider the bacterial spectrum and antibiotic susceptibility of uropathogens. Because spectrum and resistance rates may vary from time to time, area to area, and hospital to hospital, each institution must be able to provide its own local evaluation. On the other hand, antibiotics also frequently are prescribed empirically in situations in which patients do not want to wait for the results of the susceptibility testing because of their highly bothersome symptoms (eg, acute uncomplicated cystitis) [7].

Bacterial spectrum and antimicrobial resistance in urinary tract infections

Uncomplicated urinary tract infection

In uncomplicated UTIs, *Escherichia coli* is the most common pathogen, typically being isolated from more than 80% of outpatients with acute uncomplicated cystitis across various regions of the world [7]. *Staphylococcus saprophyticus* accounts for 5% to 15% of these infections and is especially prevalent in younger women who have cystitis. Causative pathogens in the remaining 5% to 10% of cases include aerobic gram-negative rods, such as *Klebsiella* and *Proteus* spp, and enterococci. The range of pathogens associated with acute uncomplicated pyelonephritis is similar to that seen in acute uncomplicated cystitis [8].

The North American Urinary Tract Infection Collaborative Alliance study from 2003 and 2004 determined resistance rates in *E coli*. Resistance to ampicillin was 38%, 21% to trimethroprim/sulfamethoxazole, 1% to nitrofurantoin, and 6% to ciprofloxacin [9]. The ARESC Project, an international surveillance study that involved nine countries in Europe and Brazil, monitored antimicrobial susceptibility of uropathogens from 2004 to 2006. The aim of the study was to rank the current usefulness of drugs used in the therapy of this condition [10]; 3018 uropathogens, including 2315 *E coli* pathogens (76.7%), 322 other gram-negative pathogens (10.7%), and 406 gram-positive pathogens (13.5%) were evaluated. Susceptibility in *E coli* was less common towards ampicillin (mean 41.1%; range 32.6%–60.8%), cotrimoxazole (70.5%; 54.5%–87.7%), and cefuroxime (81.0%; 74.5%–91.3%). Ciprofloxacin susceptibility was 91.3%, but the figures for Spain and Italy were substantially lower (88.1% and 87.0%, respectively). Fosfomycin, mecillinam, and nitrofurantoin were the agents with the highest susceptibility rates (98.1%, 95.8%; and 95.2%, respectively).

* Corresponding author.
E-mail address: wagenlehner@aol.com (F.M.E. Wagenlehner).

Complicated urinary tract infection

The bacterial spectrum of complicated, nosocomial UTI is much more heterogeneous and comprises a wide range of gram-negative and -positive species. In the latest report from the SENTRY antimicrobial surveillance program 2000, the bacterial spectrum of hospitalized urologic patients in North America consisted of 47% *E coli*, 13% *Enterococcus* spp, 11% *Klebsiella* spp, 8% *Pseudomonas* spp, 5% *Proteus mirabilis*, 4% *Enterobacter* spp, and 3% *Citrobacter* spp (less frequently isolated species not mentioned) [11]. Antibiotic resistance in *E coli* for ampicillin was 37%, 4% for ciprofloxacin, and 23% for trimethoprim/sulfamethoxazole; in *Pseudomonas aeruginosa* resistance for ciprofloxacin was 29%. Vancomycin resistance in *Enterococcus* spp was 7%, and the presence of extended-spectrum β-lactamase in *E coli* was 4% and 19% in *Klebsiella* spp.

Antibiotic substances for the treatment of urinary tract infection

To affect the bacterial cell, probably all antibiotics must get into the cell. Antimicrobial substances used for the treatment of UTI can be distinguished from those that act on the bacterial DNA, those that inhibit protein synthesis, and those that inhibit peptidoglycan synthesis. The way in which urologically important antibiotics work is alluded to in the following section.

Antibiotics that act on the DNA

Fluoroquinolones act directly on the bacterial DNA. The target structures are the bacterial topoisomerases II and IV, which introduce so-called negative "supercoils" into DNA and achieve a higher order by coiling. Four molecules of the quinolone substance form a ternary complex together with topoisomerases and DNA, which causes DNA double-strand breakage [12,13].

Sulfonamides, such as sulfamethoxazole, lead to the formation of ineffective forms of tetrahydrofolate (dihydropteroic acid) from para-aminobenzoic acid and pteridine by substituting para-aminobenzoic acid. Tetrahydrofolate physiologically is further catalyzed to dihydrofolic acid (folate), which is further catalyzed into tetrahydrofolic acid by dihydrofolate-reductase.

Pyrimethamines, such as trimethoprim, competitively inhibit the bacterial dihydrofolate-reductase. Purine synthesis is inhibited [13].

Antibiotics that inhibit protein synthesis

The aminoglycosides bind irreversibly to distinct parts of the 30S and 50S subunits of the bacterial ribosomes. Consequently, the amino acid translocation is inhibited by preventing the binding of elongation factor G. The elongation stage in bacterial translation is inhibited [13]. Oxazolidinones bind to the 23S rRNA of the 50S subunit of the bacterial ribosomes and inhibit the formation of the 70S initiation complex. The initiation stage of bacterial translation is inhibited [13].

Antibiotics that inhibit peptidoglycan synthesis

β-Lactams inhibit the last stage of peptidoglycan synthesis. They bind to penicillin-binding proteins (PBP), which act as enzymes (eg, transpeptidases, carboxypeptidases, and endopeptidases) in the formation and preservation of parts of the bacterial cell wall. The affinity of distinct penicillins for certain PBPs might be different. Penicillins inhibit the process of cross-linking of the long polysaccharide chains by short polypeptides. They are analogous substrates of the acyl-D-alanyl-D-alanine moieties and acylate transpeptidases. Consequently, the peptidoglycan wall is weakened [13]. The glycopeptide antibiotics bind to the acyl-D-alanyl-D-alanine moieties and inhibit the process of transglycosilation of the peptidoglycan wall [13].

Fosfomycin acts as an analog of phosphoenolpyruvate and forms a covalent bond with the active site cysteine residue (Cys 115) of UDP-N-acetylglucosamine enolpyruvyltransferase (MurA), which is a key enzyme of peptidoglycan synthesis [14]. It inhibits cell wall synthesis other than β-lactam antibiotics.

Mechanisms of antibiotic resistance in uropathogens

Antibiotic resistance is defined if bacteria can still grow under achievable therapeutic concentrations of antibiotic substances at the site of infection. Resistance is classified into (1) primary or inherent resistance of bacteria if bacteria are constitutively resistant against an antibacterial substance and (2) secondary or acquired resistance if resistance emerges in intrinsically susceptible bacteria. Epidemiologically important is transferable resistance located on plasmids (extrachromosomal autonomous mobile genetic element transferable to other cells) or transposons (chromosomal mobile genetic element transposable to plasmids or other chromosomal sites).

Alterations of permeability and efflux mechanisms

Intrinsic resistance of gram-negative bacteria against macrolides is caused by impermeability of the outer membrane to these hydrophilic compounds. *Enterococcus* spp show decreased permeability toward aminoglycosides and are intrinsically low level resistant to aminoglycosides. On the other hand, permeability can be altered by altered production of outer membrane proteins (eg, *E coli*), leading to decreased susceptibility to fluoroquinolones or β-lactam antibiotics.

Efflux mechanisms potentially can pump antibiotic substances, such as quinolones or tetracyclines, out of the cell. Thus far, five superfamilies of efflux transport systems are known: ATP-binding cassette (ABC), major facilitator superfamily (MFS), resistance-nodulation division (RND), small multidrug resistance (SMR), and multidrug and toxic compound extrusion (MATE) families. Efflux systems are responsible for low-level resistance and may promote selection of mutations responsible for higher level resistance [15].

A powerful efflux mechanism in *Pseudomonas* spp is one constitutively produced system (MexAB-OprM: RND superfamily) that generates intrinsic resistance against most β-lactams, quinolones, tetracycline, chloramphenicol, trimethoprim, and sulfamethoxazole. On the other side, nonconstitutive systems (ie, MexCD-OprJ, MexEF-OprN) can be expressed by mutation. In other species, such as *Staphylococcus aureus*, coagulase-negative staphylococci, or *Citrobacter freundii*, efflux is also an important mechanism of clinical resistance against quinolones [16–19].

Alterations of target structures

Target structures can be altered by mutations, acquisition of genetic material, or inactivation of antibiotics by enzymatic modification [13].

Mutations

Fluoroquinolone resistance is mediated by target modifications (DNA gyrase and/or topoisomerase IV) and decreased intracellular accumulation [16]. Although in gram-negative bacteria (eg, *E coli*) the DNA-gyrase is the primary target, in gram-positive bacteria (eg, *S aureus*) topoisomerase IV is the primary target for some but not all quinolones [17]. With clinically relevant concentrations, newer quinolones such as moxifloxacin and gemifloxacin inhibit both targets—the DNA-gyrase and topoisomerase IV.

Ampicillin resistance in enterococci is associated with overproduction of a low-affinity PBP, which is called PBP-5. High-level ampicillin resistance in *Enterococcus faecium* is associated with intrinsic overproduction of a modified PBP-5 that further lowers the penicillin-binding capability [20]. Vancomycin resistance in enterococci is caused by the manufacture of a peptidoglycan side chain from D-alanyl-D-lactate, which is incorporated into the peptidoglycan cell wall instead of the vancomycin target D-alanyl-D-alanyl. The D-alanyl-D-lactate chain shows dramatically lowered affinity to vancomycin. Vancomycin resistance is conferred by five genes located on a transposable element [21].

Acquisition of genetic material

Resistance to TMP/SMZ arises from various mechanisms that involve enzyme alteration, cellular impermeability, enzyme overproduction, inhibitor modification, or loss of binding capacity. The mechanism of greatest clinical importance is the production of plasmid-encoded, trimethoprim-resistant forms of dihydrofolate reductase [22–24]. Resistance in methicillin-resistant *S aureus* is mediated by an additional PBP-2a, which has unusually low affinity for all β-lactam antibiotics. PBP-2 and PBP-2a belong to a family of bifunctional proteins with an N-terminal transglycosylase and C-terminal transpeptidase domain. In case of blockage of PBP-2 by β-lactam antibiotics, PBP-2a takes over the enzymatic activity. PBP-2a is encoded by a *mecA*-gen that has been incorporated into the chromosomal DNA of *S aureus* and coagulase-negative staphylococci strains [25].

Inactivation of antibiotics

β-Lactamases are enzymes produced by bacteria that inactivate β-lactam antibiotics by cleavage of the β-lactam ring. More than 200 different enzymes have been identified thus far, and the substrates comprise penicillins, cephalosporins, or other β-lactam antibiotics. Resistance to penicillin is mediated by a penicillinase that hydrolyses the β-lactam ring of penicillin. More than 90% of *S aureus* isolates are penicillinase producers. This resistance can be overcome with penicillinase-stable penicillins, such as oxacillin [25]. A frequent resistance mechanism in *E coli* and *Proteus* spp is production of TEM-1, a plasmid-mediated β-lactamase that is inhibitor resistant [26]. It confers resistance in strains that have acquired the resistance plasmid (eg, to ampicillin and ampicillin/sulbactam).

The SHV-1 β-lactamase of *Klebsiella pneumoniae* and the K1 β-lactamase of *Klebsiella oxytoca* are chromosomally encoded but inhibitor sensitive [27]. It encodes intrinsic resistance in all *Klebsiella* strains, for example, to ampicillin but not to ampicillin/sulbactam. *Enterobacter* spp possess a chromosomally encoded ampC β-lactamase that inactivates penicillins and cephalosporins and is not inhibitor sensitive. Resistance, however, results only if the β-lactamase is hyperproduced. Ampicillin is a strong inducer of this enzyme. Mezlocillin is less suitable to induce hyperproduction of this β-lactamase [28].

The genus *Citrobacter* comprises such species (*Citrobacter freundii* group) that behave like *Enterobacter* spp and those that produce other less extended β-lactamases (*Citrobacter koseri/diversus*). In *Proteus* spp, a wide diversity of β-lactamases can be produced, serving as a possible β-lactamase–encoding reservoir [28,29]. Plasmid-encoded, extended-spectrum β-lactamase production is important in *K pneumoniae*, *E coli*, *Proteus* spp, and *C diversus*. Other resistances, such as aminoglycoside and trimethoprim-sulfamethoxazole resistance, are often cotransferred on the same plasmid [30].

Enterobacter spp, *C freundii*, *Serratia* spp, *K oxytoca*, *M morganii,* and *Providencia* spp possess a chromosomally encoded β-lactamase that can be induced to hyperproduction by mutation or depression [31]. This hyperproduced β-lactamase also causes a resistance phenotype, comparable to extended-spectrum β-lactamase, although no extended-spectrum β-lactamase is produced. Other inactivating enzymes can inactivate aminoglycosides or macrolides. The expression of a bifunctional aminoglycoside inactivating enzyme, 6′-N-aminoglycoside acetyltransferrase-2′-O-aminoglycoside phosphotransferase, is the most important mechanism of high-level aminoglycoside resistance in *Staphylococcus* spp and *Enterococcus* spp [32]. Enterococci are intrinsically low-level resistant; in the case of high-level resistance, aminoglycoside combination therapy would be ineffective.

Among *Enterobacteriaceae,* combinations of gentamicin-modifying enzymes are common. In *Pseudomonas* spp the combination of gentamicin-modifying enzymes and decreased permeability is common [33]. Bacteria exhibit an enormous repertoire of different resistance mechanisms. Unspecific mechanisms, such as reduced permeability or efflux, alter the tolerance to antibiotic substances less than specific mechanisms, such as inactivation of the antibiotic. The antibiotic spectrum targeted is much more extensive, however. On the other hand, unspecific mechanisms also can be induced by nonantibiotic substances, such as salicylates. Low-level resistance can be conferred and give bacteria a selection advantage.

Therapy of uncomplicated urinary tract infection

The results of the studies performed in the field of uncomplicated UTI show that antibiotic substances classically used for the treatment of uncomplicated UTI, such as cotrimoxazole, fluoroquinolones, and aminopenicillins, lose their effectiveness because of increasing resistance. Ideal substances are those with low resistance rates used exclusively for this indication, such as fosfomycin tromethamine, nitrofurantoin, and pivmecillinam.

Fosfomycin

Fosfomycin tromethamine is the oral applicable salt of fosfomycin. Fosfomycin (cis-(1R,2S)-epoxypropylphosphonic acid) is an oxirane antibiotic unrelated to other substances and is produced as a secondary metabolite by *Streptomyces* and *Pseudomonas* spp [14]. (S)-2-hydroxypropylphosphonic acid epoxidase catalyzes the epoxide ring closure of (S)-2-hydroxypropylphosphonic acid to form fosfomycin in an iron-redox mechanism [34]. Hydroxypropylphosphonic acid epoxidase represents a new subfamily of non-haem mononuclear iron enzymes that respond to its substrates with a conformational change that protects the radical-based intermediates formed during catalysis [35]. Fosfomycin is active against gram-positive and -negative bacteria but shows decreased activity against *Morganella morganii*, *Proteus vulgaris*, *P aeruginosa,* and *E faecium*. Despite many years of use, fosfomycin continues to be characterized by a low incidence of *E coli*–resistant strains (1%–3%) worldwide [36]. Fosfomycin trometamol has retained its activity against quinolone-resistant strains of *E coli,* and cross-resistance with other classes of antimicrobial agents is currently not a problem [37]. It is less active against coagulase-negative staphylococci. A meta-analysis of 2048 patients showed that overall single-dose therapy with fosfomycin trometamol exhibits equivalent results as short-term therapy with comparative agents, however [38].

Fosfomycin trometamine has approximately 40% oral bioavailability [39], and urine recovery is approximately 40% [40].

Nitrofurantoin

Nitrofurantoin belongs to the nitroheterocyclic compounds. The nitrogroup coupled onto the heterocyclic furan ring represents the proper site of effect. The nitrogroup is inactive and must be activated by microbial nitroreductases after penetration into the microbial cell [41]. Nitrofurantoin interferes with carbohydrate metabolism. The antibacterial activity is generally weak, but in urine the activity against *E coli* and some other enterobacteria, such as like *Klebsiella* spp and *Enterobacter* spp, is sufficient in the treatment of uncomplicated UTI. There is no activity against *Proteus* spp or *P aeruginosa*. Low levels of resistance to nitrofurantoin among uropathogens (*E coli* <2%) has revived interest in this agent. In women at risk for infection with resistant bacteria or in the setting of a high prevalence of TMP-SMX–resistant uropathogens, nitrofurantoin also can be used. Its use for the empiric treatment of uncomplicated cystitis is supportable from a public health perspective in an attempt to decrease uropathogen resistance because it does not share cross-resistance with more commonly prescribed antimicrobial agents [42], but short-term therapy is not well established with nitrofurantoin [43]. It is also less active against gram-negative pathogens other than *E coli*. Urinary excretion is 40% [40].

In a multicenter clinical trial, single-dose fosfomycin tromethamine, 3 g, was compared with a 7-day course of nitrofurantoin monohydrate/macrocrystal, 100 mg, for the treatment of acute uncomplicated lower UTI in female patients [44]. Seven hundred forty-nine patients were enrolled in the study (375 received fosfomycin and 374 received nitrofurantoin). Overall, 94% of pretreatment isolates were susceptible to fosfomycin and 83% were susceptible to nitrofurantoin. Bacteriologic cure rates at 5 to 11 days after initiation of treatment were 78% and 86% for fosfomycin and nitrofurantoin, respectively ($P = .02$). 1 week after treatment they were 87% and 81% for fosfomycin and nitrofurantoin, respectively ($P = .17$). Clinical success rate (cure and improvement) was higher than 80% in both treatment groups. Bacteriologic and clinical cure rates were comparable in both treatment groups [44].

Pivmecillinam

Pivmecillinam is a unique β-lactam antimicrobial agent that has been used for the treatment of acute uncomplicated UTI for more than 20 years. Pivmecillinam is the pro-drug (ester) of mecillinam with specific and high activity against gram-negative organisms such as *E coli* and other *Enterobacteriaceae*. Mecillinam is an amidine derivative of the penicillin group. Pivmecillinam is also well absorbed orally [45]. Since its introduction it has been used widely for the treatment of acute uncomplicated cystitis, primarily in the Nordic countries. The level of resistance has remained low; approximately less than 2% of *E coli* community isolates are resistant to mecillinam [46]. A comparative study (pivmecillinam versus norfloxacin) showed similar outcomes with 7 days of pivmecillinam, 200 mg, twice daily or 3 days of norfloxacin, 400 mg, twice daily when pooling bacteriologic outcomes from two studies [47]. The in vitro minimal inhibitory concentration for *S saprophyticus* is 8 to 64 mg/L, so these bacteria are considered resistant. The cure rates for this organism were reported between 73% and 92%, however. Pivmecillinam can be considered effective for treatment of cystitis caused by *S saprophyticus* [47].

Nicolle and colleagues [48] evaluated the efficacy of a 3-day regimen of pivmecillinam, 400 mg, twice daily versus norfloxacin, 400 mg, twice daily in 954 premenopausal women with symptoms of acute cystitis. Bacteriologic cure at early posttherapy follow-up was achieved in 75% of patients who took pivmecillinam and 91% of patients who took norfloxacin ($P < .001$). Clinical cure/improvement 4 days after initiation of therapy was observed in 95% of women who received pivmecillinam and 96% who received norfloxacin ($P = .39$). In women younger than 50 years, early clinical cure rates were 84% for pivmecillinam and 88% for norfloxacin ($P = .11$). Adverse effects were similar for both regimens, and there was no evidence of the emergence of increasing resistance with therapy. The authors concluded that short-course therapy with norfloxacin was superior to that with pivmecillinam in terms of bacteriologic outcome; however, clinical outcome in young women was comparable [48].

Therapy of complicated urinary tract infection

In most studies about complicated UTI, increasing rates of antibiotic resistance were found with specific species such as *E coli, P aeruginosa, Klebsiella spp, Enterobacter spp*, enterococci, and staphylococci. Extended-spectrum β-lactamases that produce *E coli* and *K pneumoniae* rapidly increase and may cause significant clinical problems in the treatment of UTI [49,50]. Although from a hygienic point of view they are regarded as not as dangerous as plasmid-encoded β-lactamases, species that produce chromosomally encoded β-lactamases also pose significant clinical problems for empiric antibiotic therapy.

Antibiotic substances with novel mode of action and effective against gram-negative pathogens are scarce. Glycylcyclines may be a new development forward; however, the currently marketed drug tigecycline is not aimed for treatment of UTI because of limited urinary excretion. In the light of these developments, old established substances, such as polymyxins, chloramphenicol, tetracycline, and temocillin, regain interest in situations in which multiply antibiotic-resistant pathogens appear. On the other hand, carbapenems still retained their activity in most of the uropathogens and are currently widely developed for treatment of complicated UTI.

Carbapenems

Carbapenems are currently available only intravenously because they are unstable, especially in gastric juice or intestinal juice. The available carbapenems are currently classified by different criteria. The classification by groups can follow the bacterial spectrum as in other antibiotic classes [51]. According to that classification, ertapenem is the sole representative of the first group and imipenem and meropenem are the representatives of the second group, which are currently licensed in Europe. Carbapenems are active against gram-positive and -negative pathogens and anaerobic pathogens. Carbapenems maintain antibacterial efficacy against most β-lactamase–producing organisms. This stability against serine-β-lactamases is caused by the trans-1-hydroxyethyl substituent and its unique juxtaposition to the β-lactam carbonyl group [52]. The stability encompasses extended spectrum-β-lactamases and AmpC β-lactamases; however, it does not extend to metallo-β-lactamases.

The group one parenteral carbapenem ertapenem has good gram-negative activity, excluding *P aeruginosa*. It is also not active against methicillin-resistant *S aureus* and enterococci. It contains a 1β-methyl substituent that reduces hydrolysis of

the β-lactam group by the renal dihydropeptidase I. It further contains a meta-substituted benzoic acid substituent, which increases the molecular weight and lipophilicity of the substance, and a carboxylic acid moiety, which results in a net negative charge. This results in a high protein binding that leads to a longer serum half-life [52]. Urinary excretion is 80% [40].

Group two parenteral carbapenems include imipenem and meropenem, which are active against many gram-positive and -negative uropathogens, excluding methicillin-resistant *S aureus, E faecium,* and vancomycin-resistant enterococci. Imipenem is hydrolysed by the renal dihydropeptidase I and is combined with the specific inhibitor cilastatin. Urinary excretion of the active imipenem is 70% if combined with cilastatin. Meropenem contains the 1β-methyl-substituent and is stable against the renal dihydropeptidase I. Compared with imipenem, it is somewhat more active against *P aeruginosa* but less active against gram-positive uropathogens. The urinary excretion of the active substance is 70% [40].

Doripenem is a new parenteral carbapenem and offers slightly more activity than meropenem against selected pathogens, including some—but not all strains—of *P aeruginosa* not susceptible to imipenem or meropenem. Doripenem is also active against gram-positive pathogens except methicillin-resistant *S aureus, E faecium,* and vancomycin-resistant enterococci. Urinary excretion is 75% and is of potential interest for the treatment of complicated UTI [53]. A large, multinational phase III study evaluated the efficacy and safety of doripenem for the treatment of complicated lower UTIs and pyelonephritis (complicated and uncomplicated) and compared it to levofloxacin [54]. A total of 753 patients were randomized. The microbiologic cure rate in the test of cure population was 82.1% for doripenem and 83.4% for levofloxacin. The clinical cure rate in the test of cure population was 95.1% for doripenem and 90.2% for levofloxacin. Doripenem was microbiologically and clinically effective and therapeutically noninferior to levofloxacin in this study for the treatment of complicated UTIs and was generally safe and well tolerated [54].

Orally active 1β-methylcarbapenems have been undergoing preclinical or clinical trials for years [55]. Substances CS-834, L-084, and DZ-2640 have been selected for further investigation [55]. CS-834 from Sankyo is the orally active prodrug of the substance R-95,867. The substance is active against gram-positive and -negative species, such as *S aureus, E coli,* and *K pneumoniae,* but is less active against *Pseudomonas* spp and *Enterococcus* spp [56]. The 24-hour cumulative renal excretion into urine in healthy volunteers ranged from 27% to 34% [55]. L-084, which was developed by Wyeth, is the orally active prodrug of L-036. This substance exhibits excellent antibacterial activity against gram-positive and -negative species, with the exception of *P aeruginosa*. The accumulative urinary recoveries in volunteers within 24 hours ranged from 54% to 73% [55]. DZ-2640 from Dai-ichi group exhibits broad antibacterial activity, except for *P aeruginosa*. The cumulative renal recoveries in volunteers ranged between 32% and 45% [55].

Urinary excretions of the oral carbapenems are certainly not optimal but are still in the intermediate range. Exaggerated consumption of carbapenems in the future will certainly lead to the emergence of antibiotic resistance and multiresistant pathogens.

Old antibiotics

The so-called "old antibiotics," such as polymyxins, chloramphenicol, doxycycline, and temocillin, have regained interest because of the need for unrelated substances in multiply-resistant organisms. None of these substances has been investigated in adequate clinical studies for the treatment of UTI, however.

Polymyxins

The increasing incidence of infections caused by multi-drug resistant *P aeruginosa* and the fact that no new antipseudomonal agent will be available in the near future caused renewed interest in the polymyxine antibiotics. Colistin and colistimethate are the only currently available compounds [57]. Colistimethate probably is the nonactive prodrug of colistin, which reacts with phospholipid components of the cytoplasma membrane and increases cell wall permeability. It displays bactericidal activity against *P aeruginosa* and extended-spectrum β-lactamase, producing gram-negative organisms. In a study of patients who had cancer and *P aeruginosa* infections, colistin was as effective and safe as β-lactam antibiotics and fluoroquinolones [58]. Colistimethate is predominantly cleared by the renal route, but a fraction of the administered dose is converted in vivo to colistin. There are some case reports of patients with UTI treated with intravenous colistimethate and good clinical outcomes reported in up to 83%, although no clinical study has been performed [57]. Nephrotoxicity and neurotoxicity are the most common potential toxicities

with parenteral administration of colistimethate, which are probably caused by inappropriate dosing. Satisfactory safety profiles have been reported with intravenous doses of 160 mg three times daily in patients with normal renal function [57].

Chloramphenicol

Chloramphenicol is active against gram-positive and -negative pathogens, with the exception of *P aeruginosa*. Resistance in enterobacteria has decreased over the last 15 years, probably because of restricted usage. Renal excretion amounts to 90%. Severe side effects have been reported, including hematologic disturbances, gastrointestinal effects, Gray syndrome, and neurologic effects [40].

Tetracycline

Doxycycline is the best orally resorbed tetracycline. Doxycycline exhibits good activity against most gram-positive bacteria, variable activity against gram-negative pathogens, and no activity against *P aeruginosa*, *Proteus* spp, and *Serratia marcescens*. Urinary recovery rates after intravenous and oral application are 70% and 40%, respectively [40].

Temocillin

Temocillin is a semisynthetic parenteral penicillin that exhibits increased stability against β-lactamases and is active against extended-spectrum β-lactamase–producing organisms. The 24-hour urinary recovery rate was between 66% and 74% of the administered doses (0.5–2 g) in volunteers [59].

Antibiotics active against otherwise resistant gram-positive uropathogens

Daptomycin and linezolid are active exclusively against gram-positive uropathogens, such as enterococci and methicillin-susceptible and -resistant staphylococci. In one study, 529 isolates of uropathogens that caused complicated UTIs were tested against daptomycin and linezolid; no resistant strain was detected [60].

Daptomycin

Daptomycin is a semisynthetic lipopeptide antibiotic with a high specificity for gram-positive bacteria [61,62]. Daptomycin apparently acts via the dissipation of the bacterial membrane potential and has a rapid concentration-dependent bactericidal activity [62]. Daptomycin showed in vitro activity superior to that of vancomycin against methicillin-resistant *S aureus*, methicillin-sensitive

S aureus, methicillin-resistant *Staphylococcus epidermidis,* and vancomycin-resistant enterococci and comparable activity against vancomycin-susceptible *E faecalis* and streptococci [62]. Daptomycin is administered intravenously, serum half-life averaged 8.5 hours, protein binding is approximately 90%, and urinary excretion is 80%, 66% of which is as active drug. Tolerability data are available for 285 patients from two multicenter, randomized phase II trials who received 2 mg/kg every 24 hours for up to 25 days or 3 mg/kg every 12 hours for up to 34 days. Daptomycin was well tolerated at these dosages with no evidence of drug-related toxicity [63]. A series of single- and repeated-dose studies in rodents, dogs, and monkeys demonstrated that the skeletal muscle is the most sensitive target organ for toxicity of daptomycin. The severity of microscopic lesions was dose dependent but did not progress with extended treatment (up to 6 months) and was completely and rapidly reversible upon cessation of dosing [62].

Linezolid

Linezolid is a member of the oxazolidinone class synthetic antibacterial agents that inhibit bacterial protein synthesis through a unique mechanism. In contrast to other inhibitors of protein synthesis, linezolid acts early in translation by preventing the formation of a functional initiation complex [64]. Linezolid is rapidly absorbed after oral dosing with an absolute bioavailability of approximately 100%. Serum half-life is approximately 5.5 hours, and protein binding is approximately 31% [65,66]. Approximately 35% of a 500-mg dose of ^{14}C-linezolid was excreted in urine as the parent drug and 50% as the two major metabolites.

In one study, urinary bactericidal titers of a single oral dose of 600 mg linezolid or 500 mg ciprofloxacin were measured in volunteers [67]. The urinary bactericidal titers of linezolid against gram-positive uropathogens, regardless of their methicillin and fluoroquinolone resistance, could be obtained for at least 12 hours and were comparable to those of ciprofloxacin in fluoroquinolone-susceptible strains, whereas there were no significant urinary bactericidal titers of ciprofloxacin in fluoroquinolone-resistant strains. The urinary bactericidal titers of linezolid have shown that with an oral dose of 600 mg linezolid twice daily, urinary bactericidal activity against gram-positive uropathogens with minimal inhibitory concentration ranges of 1 to 2 mg/L can be expected throughout the complete therapeutic interval [67].

Summary

Antibiotic resistance is an increasing problem in urologic practice. Uncomplicated and complicated—especially nosocomial—uropathogens may exhibit resistance to multiple antibiotics and pose problems for empiric therapy. To choose the right antibiotic for empiric therapy, it is necessary to consider the bacterial spectrum and antibiotic susceptibility of the uropathogens. Each institution must conduct its own local and recent evaluation. To combat the development of antibiotic resistance, a basic understanding of antibiotic action and resistance mechanisms is helpful. In the future, the rate of antibiotic resistance possibly will continue to increase. Strategies to decrease this trend, such as antibiotic policies, must be developed and incorporated in urologic practice.

References

[1] Bouza E, San Juan R, Munoz P, et al. A European perspective on nosocomial urinary tract infections. I. Report on the microbiology workload, etiology and antimicrobial susceptibility (ESGNI-003 study). European Study Group on Nosocomial Infections. Clin Microbiol Infect 2001;7(10):523–31.

[2] Foxman B. Epidemiology of urinary tract infections: incidence, morbidity, and economic costs. Am J Med 2002;113(Suppl 1A):5S–13S.

[3] Maki DG, Tambyah PA. Engineering out the risk for infection with urinary catheters. Emerg Infect Dis 2001;7(2):342–7.

[4] Ruden H, Gastmeier P, Daschner FD, et al. Nosocomial and community-acquired infections in Germany: summary of the results of the First National Prevalence Study (NIDEP). Infection 1997;25(4):199–202.

[5] Wagenlehner FM, Niemetz A, Dalhoff A, et al. Spectrum and antibiotic resistance of uropathogens from hospitalized patients with urinary tract infections: 1994–2000. Int J Antimicrob Agents 2002; 19(6):557–64.

[6] Elhanan G, Sarhat M, Raz R. Empiric antibiotic treatment and the misuse of culture results and antibiotic sensitivities in patients with community-acquired bacteraemia due to urinary tract infection. J Infect 1997;35(3):283–8.

[7] Gupta K, Hooton TM, Stamm WE. Increasing antimicrobial resistance and the management of uncomplicated community-acquired urinary tract infections. Ann Intern Med 2001;135(1):41–50.

[8] Talan DA, Stamm WE, Hooton TM, et al. Comparison of ciprofloxacin (7 days) and trimethoprim-sulfamethoxazole (14 days) for acute uncomplicated pyelonephritis in women: a randomized trial. JAMA 2000;283(12):1583–90.

[9] Zhanel GG, Hisanaga TL, Laing NM, et al. Antibiotic resistance in outpatient urinary isolates: final results from the North American Urinary Tract Infection Collaborative Alliance (NAUTICA). Int J Antimicrob Agents 2005;26(5):380–8.

[10] Naber KG, Schito GC, Gualco L (on behalf of the ARESC working group). An international survey on etiology and susceptibility of uropathogens isolated from women with uncomplicated UTI: the ARESC study. In: Interscience Conference on Antimicrobial Agents and Chemotherapy (ICAAC). Chicago, IL, 2007.

[11] Gordon KA, Jones RN. Susceptibility patterns of orally administered antimicrobials among urinary tract infection pathogens from hospitalized patients in North America: comparison report to Europe and Latin America. Results from the SENTRY Antimicrobial Surveillance Program (2000). Diagn Microbiol Infect Dis 2003;45(4):295–301.

[12] Drlica K, Zhao X. DNA gyrase, topoisomerase IV, and the 4-quinolones. Microbiol Mol Biol Rev 1997;61(3):377–92.

[13] Lehn N. Mechanismen der resistenzentwicklung gegen antibiotika: epidemiologie. In: Adam D, Doerr HW, Link H, et al, editors. Die infektiologie. Berlin: Springer-Verlag; 2004. p. 82–98.

[14] McLuskey K, Cameron S, Hammerschmidt F, et al. Structure and reactivity of hydroxypropylphosphonic acid epoxidase in fosfomycin biosynthesis by a cation- and flavin-dependent mechanism. Proc Natl Acad Sci U S A 2005;102(40):14221–6.

[15] Pechere JC, Michea-Hamzhepour M, Kohler T. [Antibiotic efflux, a mechanism of multiple resistance in Pseudomonas aeruginosa]. Bull Acad Natl Med 1998;182(3):599–612 [discussion: 595–613] [in French].

[16] Piddock LJ. Mechanisms of fluoroquinolone resistance: an update 1994–1998. Drugs 1999; 58(Suppl 2):11–8.

[17] Tanaka M, Onodera Y, Uchida Y, et al. Inhibitory activities of quinolones against DNA gyrase and topoisomerase IV purified from Staphylococcus aureus. Antimicrob Agents Chemother 1997;41(11): 2362–6.

[18] Navia MM, Ruiz J, Ribera A, et al. Analysis of the mechanisms of quinolone resistance in clinical isolates of Citrobacter freundii. J Antimicrob Chemother 1999;44(6):743–8.

[19] Linde HJ, Schmidt M, Fuchs E, et al. In vitro activities of six quinolones and mechanisms of resistance in Staphylococcus aureus and coagulase-negative staphylococci. Antimicrob Agents Chemother 2001;45(5):1553–7.

[20] Fontana R, Ligozzi M, Pittaluga F, et al. Intrinsic penicillin resistance in enterococci. Microb Drug Resist 1996;2(2):209–13.

[21] Marshall CG, Wright GD. The glycopeptide antibiotic producer Streptomyces toyocaensis NRRL 15009 has both D-alanyl-D-alanine and D-alanyl-D-lactate ligases. FEMS Microbiol Lett 1997; 157(2):295–9.

[22] Burchall JJ, Elwell LP, Fling ME. Molecular mechanisms of resistance to trimethoprim. Rev Infect Dis 1982;4(2):246–54.

[23] Park H, Bradrick TD, Howell EE. A glutamine 67-histidine mutation in homotetrameric R67 dihydrofolate reductase results in four mutations per single active site pore and causes substantial substrate and cofactor inhibition. Protein Eng 1997;10(12): 1415–24.

[24] Then RL. Mechanisms of resistance to trimethoprim, the sulfonamides, and trimethoprim-sulfamethoxazole. Rev Infect Dis 1982;4(2):261–9.

[25] Livermore DM. Antibiotic resistance in staphylococci. Int J Antimicrob Agents 2000;16(Suppl 1): S3–10.

[26] Stapleton P, Wu PJ, King A, et al. Incidence and mechanisms of resistance to the combination of amoxicillin and clavulanic acid in Escherichia coli. Antimicrob Agents Chemother 1995;39(11): 2478–83.

[27] Chaves J, Ladona MG, Segura C, et al. SHV-1 beta-lactamase is mainly a chromosomally encoded species-specific enzyme in Klebsiella pneumoniae. Antimicrob Agents Chemother 2001;45(10):2856–61.

[28] Yang YJ, Livermore DM. Chromosomal beta-lactamase expression and resistance to beta-lactam antibiotics in Proteus vulgaris and Morganella morganii. Antimicrob Agents Chemother 1988;32(9): 1385–91.

[29] Bonnet R, De Champs C, Sirot D, et al. Diversity of TEM mutants in Proteus mirabilis. Antimicrob Agents Chemother 1999;43(11):2671–7.

[30] Patterson JE. Extended-spectrum beta-lactamases. Semin Respir Infect 2000;15(4):299–307.

[31] Jones RN. Resistance patterns among nosocomial pathogens: trends over the past few years. Chest 2001;119(2 Suppl):397S–404S.

[32] Culebras E, Martinez JL. Aminoglycoside resistance mediated by the bifunctional enzyme 6′-N-aminoglycoside acetyltransferase-2″-O-aminoglycoside phosphotransferase. Front Biosci 1999;4:D1–8.

[33] The Aminoglycoside Resistance Study Groups. The most frequently occurring aminoglycoside resistance mechanisms: combined results of surveys in eight regions of the world. J Chemother 1995;7(Suppl 2): 17–30.

[34] Yan F, Munos JW, Liu P, et al. Biosynthesis of fosfomycin, re-examination and re-confirmation of a unique Fe(II)- and NAD(P)H-dependent epoxidation reaction. Biochemistry 2006;45(38):11473–81.

[35] Higgins LJ, Yan F, Liu P, et al. Structural insight into antibiotic fosfomycin biosynthesis by a mononuclear iron enzyme. Nature 2005;437(7060): 838–44.

[36] Schito GC. Why fosfomycin trometamol as first line therapy for uncomplicated UTI? Int J Antimicrob Agents 2003;22(Suppl 2):79–83.

[37] Ungheri D, Albini E, Belluco G. In-vitro susceptibility of quinolone-resistant clinical isolates of *Escherichia coli* to fosfomycin trometamol. J Chemother 2002;14(3):237–40.

[38] Lecomte F, Allaert FA. Le traitement monodose de la cystite par fosfomycin trometamol: analyse de 15 essais comparatifs portant sur 2048 malades. Med Mal Infect 1996;26:338–43.

[39] Patel SS, Balfour JA, Bryson HM. Fosfomycin tromethamine: a review of its antibacterial activity, pharmacokinetic properties and therapeutic efficacy as a single-dose oral treatment for acute uncomplicated lower urinary tract infections. Drugs 1997; 53(4):637–56.

[40] Simon C, Stille W. Antibiotika-therapie in klinik und praxis. 10th edition. Stuttgart (Germany): Schattauer; 2000.

[41] Hof H. [Antimicrobial therapy with nitroheterocyclic compounds, for example, metronidazole and nitrofurantoin]. Immun Infekt 1988;16(6):220–5 [in German].

[42] Hooton TM. The current management strategies for community-acquired urinary tract infection. Infect Dis Clin North Am 2003;17(2):303–32.

[43] Warren JW, Abrutyn E, Hebel JR, et al. Guidelines for antimicrobial treatment of uncomplicated acute bacterial cystitis and acute pyelonephritis in women. Infectious Diseases Society of America (IDSA). Clin Infect Dis 1999;29(4):745–58.

[44] Stein GE. Comparison of single-dose fosfomycin and a 7-day course of nitrofurantoin in female patients with uncomplicated urinary tract infection. Clin Ther 1999;21(11):1864–72.

[45] Lancini G, Parenti F. Antibiotics: an integrated view. New York: Springer-Verlag; 1982.

[46] Graninger W. Pivmecillinam: therapy of choice for lower urinary tract infection. Int J Antimicrob Agents 2003;22(Suppl 2):73–8.

[47] Nicolle LE. Pivmecillinam in the treatment of urinary tract infections. J Antimicrob Chemother 2000;46(Suppl 1):35–9 [discussion: 63–35].

[48] Nicolle LE, Madsen KS, Debeeck GO, et al. Three days of pivmecillinam or norfloxacin for treatment of acute uncomplicated urinary infection in women. Scand J Infect Dis 2002;34(7):487–92.

[49] Livermore DM, Woodford N. The beta-lactamase threat in *Enterobacteriaceae*, *Pseudomonas* and *Acinetobacter*. Trends Microbiol 2006;14(9): 413–20.

[50] Ena J, Arjona F, Martinez-Peinado C, et al. Epidemiology of urinary tract infections caused by extended-spectrum beta-lactamase-producing *Escherichia coli*. Urology 2006;68(6):1169–74.

[51] Shah PM, Isaacs RD. Ertapenem, the first of a new group of carbapenems. J Antimicrob Chemother 2003;52(4):538–42.

[52] Hammond ML. Ertapenem: a group 1 carbapenem with distinct antibacterial and pharmacological properties. J Antimicrob Chemother 2004;53(Suppl 2):II7–9.

[53] Jones RN, Sader HS, Fritsche TR. Comparative activity of doripenem and three other carbapenems tested against gram-negative bacilli with various beta-lactamase resistance mechanisms. Diagn Microbiol Infect Dis 2005;52(1):71–4.

[54] Naber K, Redman R, Kotey P, et al. Intravenous therapy with doripenem versus levofloxacin with an option for oral step-down therapy in the treatment of complicated urinary tract infections and pyelonephritis. Presented at the 25th ICC, 17th ECCMID. Munich, March 31-April 3, 2007.

[55] Kumagai T, Tamai S, Abe T, et al. Current status of oral carbapenem development. Current Medicinal Chemistry - Anti-Infective Agents 2002;1:1–14.

[56] van Ogtrop ML. CS-834 (Sankyo). IDrugs 1999; 2(3):254–8.

[57] Li J, Nation RL, Turnidge JD, et al. Colistin: the re-emerging antibiotic for multidrug-resistant gram-negative bacterial infections. Lancet Infect Dis 2006;6(9):589–601.

[58] Hachem RY, Chemaly RF, Ahmar CA, et al. Colistin is effective in the treatment of multidrug-resistant *Pseudomonas aeruginosa* infections in cancer patients. Antimicrob Agents Chemother 2007; 51(6):1905–11.

[59] Hampel B, Feike M, Koeppe P, et al. Pharmacokinetics of temocillin in volunteers. Drugs 1985; 29(Suppl 5):99–102.

[60] Wagenlehner FM, Lehn N, Witte W, et al. In vitro activity of daptomycin versus linezolid and vancomycin against gram-positive uropathogens and ampicillin against enterococci, causing complicated urinary tract infections. Chemotherapy 2005;51(2–3):64–9.

[61] Allen NE, Hobbs JN, Alborn WE Jr. Inhibition of peptidoglycan biosynthesis in gram-positive bacteria by LY146032. Antimicrob Agents Chemother 1987; 31(7):1093–9.

[62] Snydman DR, Jacobus NV, McDermott LA, et al. Comparative in vitro activities of daptomycin and vancomycin against resistant gram-positive pathogens. Antimicrob Agents Chemother 2000;44(12): 3447–50.

[63] De Bruin MF, Tally FP. Efficacy and safety of daptomycin for the treatment of bacteremia and serious infections due to gram-positive bacteria. Presented at the 4th Decennial International Conference on Nosocomial and Healthcare-Associated Infections. Atlanta, GA, March 5–9, 2000.

[64] Shinabarger D. Mechanism of action of the oxazolidinone antibacterial agents. Expert Opin Investig Drugs 1999;8(8):1195–202.

[65] Conte JE Jr, Golden JA, Kipps J, et al. Intrapulmonary pharmacokinetics of linezolid. Antimicrob Agents Chemother 2002;46(5):1475–80.

[66] MacGowan AP. Pharmacokinetic and pharmacodynamic profile of linezolid in healthy volunteers and

patients with gram-positive infections. J Antimicrob
Chemother 2003;51(Suppl 2):II17–25.

[67] Wagenlehner FM, Wydra S, Onda H, et al. Concentrations in plasma, urinary excretion, and bactericidal activity of linezolid (600 milligrams) versus those of ciprofloxacin (500 milligrams) in healthy volunteers receiving a single oral dose. Antimicrob Agents Chemother 2003;47(12):3789–94.

ELSEVIER
SAUNDERS

Urol Clin N Am 35 (2008) 81–89

UROLOGIC
CLINICS
of North America

Chronic Prostatitis/Chronic Pelvic Pain Syndrome

Michel A. Pontari, MD

Department of Urology, Temple University School of Medicine,
3401 North Broad Street, Zone C, Suite 330, Philadelphia, PA 19140, USA

In the 20th century, the term "prostatitis" traditionally referred to inflammation in the prostate, often attributed to infection. Prostatitis in this century usually refers to a chronic pain syndrome for which the presence of inflammation and involvement of the prostate are not always certain.

Definition and classification

The traditional classification of prostatitis, proposed by Drach and colleagues [1] in 1978, included acute prostatitis, chronic bacterial prostatitis, chronic nonbacterial prostatitis, and prostatodynia. A more recent classification was adopted in 1995 after a National Institutes of Health (NIH)-sponsored consensus conference and expands the classification (Table 1) [2]. In the current system, Category I and II reflect acute and chronic bacterial prostatitis, respectively. Together, both account for no more than 5% to 10% of all cases [3]. These cases are clearly associated with bacterial infection and will have a urine culture that grows uropathogens. Acute prostatitis is characterized by the sudden onset of fever and dysuria, whereas chronic bacterial prostatitis typically involves relapsing episodes of urinary tract infections, usually with the same organism seen on urine cultures. These patients are usually asymptomatic between infections. Category IV refers to asymptomatic inflammatory prostatitis that is diagnosed incidentally during a work up for infertility, an elevated prostate-specific antigen (PSA), or benign prostatic hyperplasia (BPH). The recent MTOPS study linked prostate inflammation to increased progression of symptoms or

urinary retention in a cohort of BPH subjects [4,5], so the idea that type IV is asymptomatic may be outdated. More accurately it may reflect lower urinary tract symptoms without pelvic pain, but this has not been unequivocally established.

Category III, known as chronic prostatitis/chronic pelvic pain syndrome (CP/CPPS), constitutes the vast majority (more than 90%) of cases, and is divided into IIIA and IIIB. IIIA refers to the presence of white blood cells in semen, after prostate massage urine specimen (VB3), or expressed prostatic secretion (EPS). This corresponds to the previously used classification of nonbacterial prostatitis. Category IIIB is comparable to the formerly used term "prostatodynia," and refers to patients with pelvic pain but no evidence of inflammation on semen, VB3, or EPS. The symptom that distinguishes CP/CPPS from other voiding dysfunction is the presence of pain [6]. The current NIH definition of CP/CPPS is that of genitourinary pain in the absence of uropathogenic bacteria detected by standard microbiologic methods [2].

Epidemiology

To examine health care use in men with prostatitis, a review of available outpatient visit data was conducted through the Urologic Diseases in America project [7]. Physician office visit rates for patients with prostatitis listed as any diagnosis were determined from National Ambulatory Medical Care Survey data for the even years between 1992 and 2000. The age-adjusted visit rate in 2000 was 1,867 per 100,000 population, with the number of physician office visits totaling 1,795,643. Until recently, prostatitis was

E-mail address: pontarm@tuhs.temple.edu

Table 1
NIH classification of prostatitis

Category	Description/Type	
I	Acute bacterial prostatitis	
II	Chronic bacterial prostatitis	
III	Chronic prostatitis/ chronic pelvic pain syndrome	
IIIA		Inflammatory[a]
IIIB		Noninflammatory[a]
IV	Asymptomatic inflammation of the prostate	

[a] Inflammation is determined by the presence of white blood cell counts in one of the following: after prostate massage urine specimen, seminal plasma, or expressed prostatic secretions.

considered a problem only in younger men. In the NIH sponsored Chronic Prostatitis Collaborative Research Network (CPCRN) study, the mean age was 42 years old but the age range was 20 to 83 [8].

Men with CPPS suffer significant declines in quality of life. The sickness impact for chronic prostatitis is similar to scores reported in the literature for patients with myocardial infarction and Crohn's disease [9]. McNaughton-Collins and colleagues [10] used the twelve item short form health survey to evaluate the mental and physical health of CP/CPPS patients and found that the mental component summary score for CPPS patients was lower than that observed in the most severe subgroups of congestive heart failure and diabetes [11].

Men with CP/CPPS are more likely to have several other conditions. In the CPCRN study, men with CP/CPPS, as compared with age-matched controls, were six times more likely to have cardiovascular disease, five times more likely to have neurologic disease (especially vertebral disk disease), and twice as likely to have sinusitis and anxiety or depression [12]. These associations raise the question of what common abnormalities may be present in CP/CPPS and these other conditions. The most common diagnosis under cardiovascular history in the author's patients was hypertension, followed by atherosclerotic disease.

A study of prostatitis in a large managed care database found that men with prostatitis were more likely to have 35 other diagnoses, which fell under the categories of other urologic conditions

(10), unexplained somatic symptoms (19), and psychiatric conditions (4) [13]. Sexual dysfunction is also common in men with CP/CPPS. In a study of a large urban population in Austria, 2.7% of men reported a pain score of at least 4 out of 10, and in men with the most severe prostatitis symptoms, the risk of erectile dysfunction was increased 8.3 fold [14].

Etiology and pathogenesis

The etiology of CP/CPPS is unknown. Many different theories and mechanisms for the pathogenesis of prostatitis have been proposed. One question is whether the prostate inflammation is actually a source of symptoms in men with CP/CPPS. True and colleagues [15] found prostatic inflammation in only 33% of patients with CP/CPPS who underwent transperineal prostate biopsy. These findings raise the question of whether the prostate is even actually involved in the symptoms of CP/CPPS. The name "chronic pelvic pain syndrome" recognizes that the prostate may not be the sole source of discomfort, and that there may be other factors or anatomic sites involved.

Traditionally, white blood cells (WBCs) in the prostatic fluids have been studied and thought to be markers for an inflammatory process that contributes to the symptoms of prostatitis. The use of WBCs as markers of inflammation is limited for several reasons. WBCs can be found in the prostatic fluid or seminal plasma of asymptomatic men, as well as those with pelvic pain [16,17]. In addition, in symptomatic men, none of the measures of the NIH-chronic prostatitis symptom index (NIH-CPSI), including subsets for pain, urinary, and quality of life, show any correlation with WBCs in either EPS, VB3, or seminal plasma [16]. Another argument against the association between inflammation and symptoms is that category IIIB patients have symptoms but no inflammation.

Infection

The symptoms of CP/CPPS are identical to those of a true prostatic infection. Therefore, one of the most prevalent theories as to the development of symptoms in these men is that of an occult or undertreated infection. Despite the lack of an ongoing infection in men with CP/CPPS, in the NIH cohort study, there was a significantly greater self-reported history of nonspecific urethritis as compared with age-matched controls;

gonorrheal, trichomonal, and genital herpetic infections were not significantly different [12]. The NIH cohort study found no differences between cases and controls in sexual practices, including types of sexual contact and numbers of partners [12]. Controls tended to be younger at age of first intercourse. This data does not support a difference in sexual practices or frequency in men with CPPS compared with controls. However, it does not rule out and may even suggest the possibility of a sexually transmitted disease as an initial source of inflammation that in susceptible men goes on to cause chronic pain long after the initial acute infection has resolved. This is also consistent with findings from a study of over 30,000 male health professionals, in which those men reporting a history of sexually transmitted disease had 1.8-fold greater odds of a self-reported history of prostatitis [18].

Newer studies have also increasingly used molecular techniques to try to answer the question of infection in these patients. Shoskes and Shahed [19] found that performing polymerase chain reaction (PCR) on EPS detected the presence of bacterial DNA in category IIIA patients in 23 (70%) of 33 specimens, whereas culture was positive (for Gram-positive bacteria) in only 17 (51%) of 33 specimens. Only 2 of 14 category IIIB patients had bacterial DNA. Nevertheless, 13 (57%) of the total patients with bacterial DNA improved with antibiotics, while patients that lacked bacterial DNA by PCR did not improve with antibiotics. Direct comparison of PCR performed in prostate tissue, taken at the time of radical prostatectomy for prostate cancer in men with and without symptoms of chronic pelvic pain, have shown no differences in product for herpes simplex virus, cytomegalovirus, papillomavirus, nor bacterial DNA [20,21]. Using PCR on perineal biopsies from men with and without pelvic pain and no prostate cancer showed no differences in rates of positive findings for bacteria [22].

Overall, it seems unlikely that there is an ongoing acute infection. Particularly intriguing is the finding of cultures localizing uropathogenic bacteria to the prostate in 8% of asymptomatic men with CPPS, and what are considered to be nonuropathogens in 74% of asymptomatic age-matched controls [17]. This suggests that the prostate of normal asymptomatic males harbors bacteria.

Another possibility in men with symptoms is that of a dysregulation of pro- and anti-inflammatory cytokines leading to inflammation from otherwise normal prostate bacteria. There have been multiple reports of abnormal level cytokines in EPS and seminal plasma, including interleukin (IL)-8 [23], IL-10 [24] IL-1B and tumor necrosis factor (TNF)-α [25]. However, although there have been differences shown between CP/CPPS patients and controls, there has been no consistent pattern across all studies [26].

Finally, a confounding factor that has not been resolved nor even closely studied so far in CP/CPPS, is that of bacterial biofilms. Bacteria that grow in standard culture techniques are free floating so called "planktonic" bacteria. However, bacteria may also exist in biofilms, in which they form communities of surface adherent organisms embedded in extracellular matrix [27]. The biofilms certainly pose a different environment for standard antibiotics, and even may elicit cytokine responses from leukocytes [28]. What role these biofilms play in the development of prostate infections and CP/CPPS needs to be addressed in the future.

Neurologic factors

The fact that men suffering from CPPS have pain indicates some neurologic involvement, either on a local level or in the central nervous system. Therefore, one hypothesis of the etiology and pathogenesis of CPPS is that there is dysfunction of the nervous system leading to pain. Experimental evidence for central remodeling is provided by the finding that chemical irritation of rat prostate and bladder causes c-fos expression at spinal cord levels L6 and S1, along with plasma extravasation in the skin at the identical L6 and S1 dermatomes, underscoring the overlap of afferent nerve fiber distribution [29]. This corresponds in the human being to the distribution of the umbilicus to mid thigh, which is the common distribution of pain in individuals with CPPS. Retrograde labeling of both prostate and pelvic floor indicates that there are double labeled cells in the dorsal root ganglion in the lumbar and sacral cord in an animal model, indicating the close relationship neurologically between the two areas [30].

The presence of central sensitization in patients with CPPS was demonstrated by Yang and colleagues [31], who compared thermal algometry in men with CPPS and asymptomatic controls. Sensitivity to noxious heat stimuli is thought to be a reflection of central sensitization. The men with CPPS reported a higher visual analog scale to short bursts of noxious heat stimuli to the perineum, but no difference to the anterior thigh. Thus, these patients have altered sensation in the perineum when compared with controls. This is similar to other chronic pain syndromes, such as reflex sympathetic dystrophy and fibromyalgia, where patients also have heightened responses to noxious heat stimuli in areas of chronic pain, compared with controls. Similar findings were reported using capsaicin applied to the skin overlying the perineal body [32].

Psychologic factors and stress response

Psychologic factors also appear to be involved in producing symptoms in men with CP/CPPS and psychologic stress is a common finding in men with CPPS [33]. In addition to pain intensity, depressive symptoms significantly predict a worse quality of life in men with CP/CPPS than in men without [34]. Psychologic variables also affect pain perception. Pelvic pain in CP/CPPS also is dependent upon helplessness, catastrophizing, and depression [35].

Ullrich and colleagues [36] prospectively examined whether perceived stress was associated longitudinally with pain intensity and pain-related disability in a sample of men with nonbacterial prostatitis and pelvic pain. Over 200 patients with CP/CPPS completed measures of perceived stress, pain intensity, and pain-related disability 1 month after a health care visit, with a new nonbacterial prostatitis or pelvic pain diagnosis 3, 6, and 12 months later. They found that greater perceived stress during the 6 months after the health-care visit was associated with greater pain intensity ($P = .03$) and disability ($P = .003$) at 12 months, even after controlling for age, symptom duration, and pain and disability during the first 6 months. Lee and colleagues [37] recently reported on elevated levels of catecholamines in the urine of men with CPPS, compared with controls, as well as increased allostatic load. Measuring the allostatic load or stress response of a large group of patients as a correlate of symptoms and clinical course should be studied.

Genetics

Several genetic differences between men with CP/CPPS and controls have been identified. Differences in the DNA sequence or polymorphisms have been identified in the promoter regions of several cytokines. Polymorphisms in the genes or promoters for IL-10 and TNF-α

are associated with low IL-10 or TNF-α production [38]. In a recent study, significantly more men with CPPS expressed the IL-10 AA genotype compared with controls (11 of 36 or 31% versus 33 out of 272 or 12%; $P = .007$) [39]. All eight IIIA patients had the low TNF-α production genotype. There was no difference in the TNF-α genotype in the 22 IIIB patients versus 272 controls, but all eight of the IIIA patients had the low TNF-α genotype. Differences have been reported in the frequency of three alleles near the phosphoglycerate kinase (PGK) gene, between CPPS patients and controls [40]. The alleles differed in the number of short tandem repeats. The PGK1 gene in the region assessed has been found to be associated with familial prostate cancer, hypospadias, and androgen insensitivity. Another gene in the same region of the X chromosome, Xq11 to Xq13, is the androgen receptor. This finding raises the possibility of androgen insensitivity or dysfunction in the pathogenesis of CPPS.

Association with other diseases

The systemic symptoms for CP/CPPS—including fatigue, pain, disability out of proportion to physical examination, and an association with stress or psychosocial factors—are similar to those seen in other poorly explained clinical conditions, including fibromyalgia, irritable bowel syndrome, and chronic fatigue syndrome [41]. In a recent study, functional somatic syndromes and psychologic disorders were significantly more prevalent among men with CP/CPPS as compared with the general population [42]. Thus, there is a growing perception that CP/CPPS may be one manifestation of one or more of these somatic syndromes [43]. For instance, cardiovascular history is of interest in men with CPPS, given the presence of cardiac signs of autonomic neuropathy in these other poorly explained chronic diseases [44].

Evaluation

The basic principle underlying evaluation of men with CP/CPPS is to try to identify specific and hopefully treatable causes of the pelvic pain. In the majority of men, no such cause will be identified. However, it is important not to miss a possible reversible cause of the symptoms in these men. There is no accepted standard evaluation for men with CP/CPPS. Mandatory measures include a history, physical examination (including digital rectal examination and urinalysis), and urine culture [45]. In the older man with symptoms of CP/CPPS, the digital rectal exam is very important to look for prostate nodules that should prompt a biopsy to rule out prostate carcinoma. Recommended studies include the assessment of symptoms. This has been greatly facilitated by the CPCRN with the development of the NIH-CPSI, a self-administered validated symptom index [46]. Other recommended studies include some form of lower urinary tract localization studies. The evaluation of chronic prostatitis has traditionally used the Meares-Stamey four glass test (VB1, VB2, EPS, VB3) but the use of a pre- and postprostate massage urine provides similar information [47]. Another recommended investigation is determination of post-void residual urine.

There are many optional studies, as outlined in the recent summary statement by Nickel [45]. The role of imaging studies is controversial, but prostatic ultrasound may be especially helpful in the man who has pain after ejaculation, to look for lesions such as prostatic and mullerian remnant cysts. Patients with urethral discharge should have a urethral swab. Urodynamics can be used in men whose voiding symptoms are refractory to treatment. It is also important to further evaluate abnormalities in the workup and not to ascribe these findings necessarily to the CP/CPPS alone. Two examples include the findings of hematuria and an elevated PSA. Hematuria, microscopic or gross, should not be attributed solely to the prostatitis, and should be further evaluated with cystoscopy, urine cytology, and a study of the upper urinary tracts. PSA measurement is not standard in the evaluation of CP/CPPS, but is done frequently as screening for prostate cancer in men over age 40 in African American men or those with a family history, or age 50 in other individuals. PSA is slightly elevated in men with CP/CPPS as compared with asymptomatic controls [48], but not enough to account for elevated PSA greater than 4.0, which should prompt a prostate biopsy despite the presence of CP/CPPS.

Treatment of CP/CPPS

Limitations in the treatment of CP/CPPS include lack of a clear etiology to guide appropriate therapy and a dearth of randomized placebo-controlled trials for the treatments that are already being used.

Antibiotics have played a central role in the treatment of men with CP/CPPS, as many ascribed theses symptoms to infection. The results of antibiotics for treatment of CP/CPPS in controlled trials are mixed. Nickel and colleagues [49] compared levofloxacin to placebo in CP/CPPS, using both for 6 weeks. There was not a statistically significant difference in efficacy, but more patients responded to levofloxacin, as defined by a 6-point decrease in NIH-CPSI score. The CPCRN group compared ciprofloxacin to placebo in a randomized placebo-controlled trial and again found no statistically significant difference [50]. It is common to use an empiric 4 to 6 week course of antibiotics in men with CP/CPPS who are antibiotic naïve, but certainly the use of repeated courses of antimicrobials in these men is not warranted [51]. Antibiotics have also been combined with treatment for prostatic stones to treat nanobacteria, and resulted in clinically significant improvement in symptoms in a pilot study [52].

Alpha-blockers are commonly used in therapy for CP/CPPS. The CPCRN randomized clinical trial showed no significant efficacy of tamsulosin compared with placebo. However, two factors may help to explain this comparative lack of efficacy. First, patients were not alpha-blocker naïve. Second, the treatment was for only 6 weeks. A meta analysis of treatment trials of alpha-adrenergic antagonists in men with CP/CPPS indicated that combined analysis showed a significant reduction in total NIH-CPSI score or internal prostate symptom score, and that the duration of treatment needs to be at least 3-months long to see the effect [53]. Other trials have shown moderate efficacy of alpha blockers used for at least 6 weeks [54–56].

Beyond the initial treatment with antibiotic and alpha-adrenergic antagonists, there are many other medications that can be used. Standard anti-inflammatory medications may be effective. Another compound that has anti-inflammatory effect is the bioflavinoid quercetin. In a randomized placebo controlled trial, quercetin produced significant reduction in NIH-CPSI symptom scores ($P = .003$), and was generally well tolerated [57]. Pentosan polysulfate is a semi-synthetic muco-polysaccharide that may also have some anti-inflammatory properties. A recent randomized placebo-controlled trial used 900 mg by mouth every day for 16 weeks versus placebo: there was a moderate or marked clinical global improvement with PPS, 36.7%, versus placebo, 17.8%

$(P = .04)$ [58]. Standard dose therapy is 100 mg by mouth three times a day, and the dose of pentosanpolysulfate appears less important than an adequate duration of therapy, which should be at least 6 months [59]. Finasteride has also been studied for men with CP/CPPS. In patients with category IIIA prostatitis, 6 months of therapy with finasteride versus placebo resulted in a 50% improvement in global assessment in 44% of subjects on finasteride and 27% on placebo [60]. Finasteride is an attractive medication to use in older men with CP/CPPS because it also can be effective on benign prostatic hyperplasia, which can be concurrent in men with symptoms of CP/CPPS.

As the main symptom of CP/CPPS is pain, other treatments target pain specifically. Tricyclic antidepressant medications (TCA) are widely used for neuropathic pain. Tricyclics are thought to block pain by inhibiting the central neuronal reuptake of norepinephrine and serotonin, potentiating the inhibitory effect of these substances on the central pain processing receptor [61]. More recent reviews of treatment of neuropathic pain have suggested nortriptyline as first line therapy when using TCAs, given its favorable side effect profile [62]. Currently the author uses nortriptyline as a first line TCA because it may produce less sedation than amitriptyline, and many of the author's patients are relatively young and working. Starting doses are 10 mg by mouth at bedtime, working up to a maximum of 75 mg to 100 mg by mouth at bedtime. Gabapentin and pregabalin are anticonvulsants that are also effective in treating neuropathic pain. Pregabalin has recently been approved for the treatment of post herpetic neuralgia [63] and diabetic neuropathy [64], and is under study in a randomized placebo controlled trial for CP/CPPS. Finally, opioids may be needed to treat severe pain [65]. Referral to a pain center may also be helpful in cases of severe pain.

Other therapies for CP/CPPS include physical therapy and myofascial or trigger point release [66]. In a series from Stanford, pelvic floor physical therapy improved not only overall symptoms, but also specifically improved sexual dysfunction [67]. Acupuncture has also been suggested as therapy for CP/CPPS [68]. Generally, prostate specific therapies, such as microwave thermotherapy or transurethral needle ablation have demonstrated limited efficacy [69].

The most important aspect of treatment is that monotherapy is usually not successful, and multimodal therapy is usually required in these patients [70]. This includes addressing pain, voiding symptoms, and quality of life issues. This involves a combined biopsychosocial approach, which goes beyond just prescribing medications [71].

References

[1] Drach GW, Fair WR, Meares EM, et al. Classification of benign diseases associated with prostatic pain: prostatitis or prostatodynia? J Urol 1978; 120(2):266.

[2] Krieger JN, Nyberg L Jr, Nickel JC. NIH consensus definition and classification of prostatitis. JAMA 1999;282(3):236–7.

[3] de la Rosette JJ, Hubregtse MR, Meuleman EJ, et al. Diagnosis and treatment of 409 patients with prostatitis syndromes. Urology 1993;41(4):301–7.

[4] Roehrborn CG, Kaplan SA, Noble WD, et al. The impact of acute or chronic inflammation in baseline biopsy on the risk of clinical progression of BPH: Results from the MTOPS study. J Urol 2005; 173(4 Suppl):346 [abstract].

[5] Roehrborn CG. Definition of at-risk patients: baseline variables. BJU Int 2006;97(Suppl 2):7–11 [discussion: 21–2].

[6] Krieger JN, Egan KJ, Ross SO, et al. Chronic pelvic pains represent the most prominent urogenital symptoms of "chronic prostatitis.". Urology 1996; 48(5):715–21 [discussion: 721–22].

[7] McNaughton-Collins MM, Pontari MA. Prostatitis. In: Litwin MS, Saigal CS, editors. US Department of Health and Human Services, Public Health Service, National Institutes of Health, National Institute of Diabetes and Digestive and Kidney Diseases. Vol NIH Publication No. 07–5512. Washington, DC: US Government Printing Office; 2007. p. 9–42.

[8] Schaeffer AJ, Landis JR, Knauss JS, et al. Demographic and clinical characteristics of men with chronic prostatitis: the National Institutes of Health chronic prostatitis cohort study. J Urol 2002;168: 593–8 [see comment].

[9] Wenninger K, Heiman JR, Rothman I, et al. Sickness impact of chronic nonbacterial prostatitis and its correlates. J Urol 1996;155(3):965–8.

[10] Ware JE, Kosinski M, Keller SD. A twelve item short form health survey-construction of scales and preliminary tests of reliability and validity. Med Care 1996;34:220–3.

[11] McNaughton Collins M, Pontari MA, O'Leary MP, et al. Quality of life is impaired in men with chronic prostatitis: the Chronic Prostatitis Collaborative Research Network. J Gen Intern Med 2001;16(10): 656–62.

[12] Pontari MA, McNaughton-Collins M, O'Leary MP, et al. A case-control study of risk factors in men with

chronic pelvic pain syndrome. BJU Int 2005;96(4): 559–65.

[13] Clemens JQ, Meenan RT, Rosetti MCO, et al. Prevalence and risk factors for prostatitis in a managed care population. J Urol 2007;177(Suppl 4):30.

[14] Marszalek M, Wehrberger C, Hochreiter W, et al. Symptoms suggestive of chronic pelvic pain syndrome in an urban population: prevalence and associations with lower urinary tract symptoms and erectile function. J Urol 2007; 177(5):1815–9.

[15] True LD, Berger RE, Rothman I, et al. Prostate histopathology and the chronic prostatitis/chronic pelvic pain syndrome: a prospective biopsy study. J Urol 1999;162:2014–8.

[16] Schaeffer AJ, Knauss JS, Landis JR, et al. Leukocyte and bacterial counts do not correlate with severity of symptoms in men with chronic prostatitis: the National Institutes of Health Chronic Prostatitis Cohort Study. J Urol 2002;168(3):1048–53.

[17] Nickel JC, Alexander RB, Schaeffer AJ, et al. Leukocytes and bacteria in men with chronic prostatitis/chronic pelvic pain syndrome compared to asymptomatic controls. J Urol 2003;170:818–22.

[18] Collins MM, Meigs JB, Barry MJ, et al. Prevalence and correlates of prostatitis in the health professionals follow-up study cohort. J Urol 2002;167: 1363–6.

[19] Shoskes DA, Shahed AR. Detection of bacterial signal by 16S rRNA polymerase chain reaction in expressed prostatic secretions predicts response to antibiotic therapy in men with chronic pelvic pain syndrome. Tech Urol 2000;6(3):240–2.

[20] Leskinen MJ, Rantakokko-Jalava K, Manninen R, et al. Negative bacterial polymerase chain reaction (PCR) findings in prostate tissue from patients with symptoms of chronic pelvic pain syndrome (CPPS) and localized prostate cancer. Prostate 2003;55(2):105–10.

[21] Leskinen MJ, Vainionp R, Syrjnen S, et al. Herpes simplex virus, cytomegalovirus, and papillomavirus DNA are not found in patients with chronic pelvic pain syndrome undergoing radical prostatectomy for localized prostate cancer. Urology 2003;61(2): 397–401.

[22] Lee JC, Muller CH, Rothman I, et al. Prostate biopsy culture findings of men with chronic pelvic pain syndrome do not differ from those of healthy controls [see comment]. J Urol 2003;169(2):584–7 [discussion: 587–8].

[23] Hochreiter WW, Nadler RB, Koch AE, et al. Evaluation of the cytokines interleukin 8 and epithelial neutrophil activating peptide 78 as indicators of inflammation in prostatic secretions. Urology 2000; 56(6):1025–9.

[24] Miller LJ, Fischer KA, Goralnick SJ, et al. Interleukin-10 levels in seminal plasma: implications for chronic prostatitis-chronic pelvic pain syndrome. J Urol 2002;167(2 Pt 1):753–6.

[25] Nadler RB, Koch AE, Calhoun EA, et al. IL-1beta and TNF-alpha in prostatic secretions are indicators in the evaluation of men with chronic prostatitis. J Urol 2000;164(1):214–8.

[26] Pontari MA, Ruggieri MR. Mechanisms in prostatitis/chronic pelvic pain syndrome. J Urol 2004; 172(3):839–45.

[27] Costerton JW, Stewart PS, Greenberg EP. Bacterial biofilms: a common cause of persistent infections. Science 1999;284:1318–22.

[28] Leid JG, Shirtliff ME, Costerton JW, et al. Human leukocytes adhere to, penetrate, and respond to Staphylococcus aureus biofilms. Infect Immun 2002;70:6339–45.

[29] Ishigooka M, Zermann DH, Doggweiler R, et al. Similarity of distributions of spinal c-Fos and plasma extravasation after acute chemical irritation of the bladder and the prostate. J Urol 2000; 164(5):1751–6.

[30] Chen Y, Song B, Jin XY, et al. Possible mechanism of referred pain in the perineum and pelvis associated with the prostate in rats. J Urol 2005;174(6): 2405–8.

[31] Yang CC, Lee JC, Kromm BG, et al. Pain sensitization in male chronic pelvic pain syndrome: why are symptoms so difficult to treat? J Urol 2003;170(3): 823–6 [discussion: 826–7].

[32] Turini D, Beneforti P, Spinelli M, et al. Heat/burning sensation induced by topical application of capsaicin on perineal cutaneous area: new approach in diagnosis and treatment of chronic prostatitis/chronic pelvic pain syndrome? Urology 2006;67(5): 910–3.

[33] Mehik A, Hellstrom P, Sarpola A, et al. Fears, sexual disturbances and personality features in men with prostatitis: a population-based cross-sectional study in Finland. BJU Int 2001;88(1):35–8.

[34] Tripp DA, Curtis Nickel J, Landis JR, et al. Predictors of quality of life and pain in chronic prostatitis/chronic pelvic pain syndrome: findings from the National Institutes of Health Chronic Prostatitis Cohort Study. BJU Int 2004;94(9):1279–82.

[35] Tripp DA, Nickel JC, Wang Y, et al. Catastrophizing and pain-contingent rest predict patient adjustment in men with chronic prostatitis/chronic pelvic pain syndrome. J Pain 2006;7(10):697–708.

[36] Ullrich PM, Turner JA, Ciol M, et al. Stress is associated with subsequent pain and disability among men with nonbacterial prostatitis/pelvic pain. Ann Behav Med 2005;30(2):112–8.

[37] Lee J, Nickel JC, Downey J, et al. Chronic Pelvic Pain Syndrome patients show evidence of allostatic overload. J Urol 2006;175(Suppl):30.

[38] Turner DM, Williams DM, Sankaran D, et al. An investigation of polymorphism in the interleukin-10 gene promoter. Eur J Immunogenet 1997;24:1–8.

[39] Shoskes DA, Albakri Q, Thomas K, et al. Cytokine polymorphisms in men with chronic prostatitis/chronic pelvic pain syndrome: association with

diagnosis and treatment response. J Urol 2002; 168(1):331–5.

[40] Riley DE, Krieger JN. X Chromosomal short tandem repeat polymorphisms near the phosphoglycerate kinase gene in men with chronic prostatitis. Biochim Biophys Acta 2002;1586(1):99–107.

[41] Wessely S, Nimnuan C, Sharpe M. Functional somatic syndromes: one or many? [see comment] Lancet 1999;354(9182):936–9.

[42] Potts J, Moritz N, Everson D, et al. Chronic abacterial prostatitis: a functional somatic syndrome? J Urol 2001;165(Suppl):25.

[43] Potts JM. Chronic pelvic pain syndrome: a non-prostatocentric perspective. World J Urol 2003;21:54–6.

[44] Yoshiuchi K, Quigley KS, Ohashi K, et al. Use of time-frequency analysis to investigate temporal patterns of cardiac autonomic response during head-up tilt in chronic fatigue syndrome. Auton Neurosci 2004;113(1–2):55–62.

[45] Nickel JC. Clinical evaluation of the man with chronic prostatitis/chronic pelvic pain syndrome. Urology 2002;60(Suppl 6):20–2 [discussion: 22–3].

[46] Litwin MS, McNaughton-Collins M, Fowler FJ Jr, et al. The National Institutes of Health chronic prostatitis symptom index: development and validation of a new outcome measure. Chronic Prostatitis Collaborative Research Network. J Urol 1999;162(2): 369–75.

[47] Nickel JC, Shoskes D, Wang Y, et al. How does the pre-massage and post-massage 2-glass test compare to the Meares-Stamey 4-glass test in men with chronic prostatitis/chronic pelvic pain syndrome? J Urol 2006;176(1):119–24.

[48] Nadler RB, Collins MM, Propert KJ, et al. Prostate-specific antigen test in diagnostic evaluation of chronic prostatitis/chronic pelvic pain syndrome. Urology 2006;67(2):337–42.

[49] Nickel JC, Downey J, Clark J, et al. Levofloxacin for chronic prostatitis/chronic pelvic pain syndrome in men: a randomized placebo-controlled multicenter trial. Urology 2003;62(4):614–7.

[50] Alexander RB, Propert KJ, Schaeffer AJ, et al. Ciprofloxacin or tamsulosin in men with chronic prostatitis/chronic pelvic pain syndrome: a randomized, double-blind trial [see comment] [summary for patients in Ann Intern Med. 2004 Oct 19;141(8):I8; PMID: 15492335]. Ann Intern Med 2004;141(8): 581–9.

[51] Shoskes DA. Use of antibiotics in chronic prostatitis syndromes. Can J Urol 2001;8(Suppl 1):24–8.

[52] Shoskes DA, Thomas KD, Gomez E. Anti-nanobacterial therapy for men with chronic prostatitis/chronic pelvic pain syndrome and prostatic stones: preliminary experience. J Urol 2005;173(2):474–7.

[53] Yang G, Wei Q, Li H, et al. The effect of alpha-adrenergic antagonists in chronic prostatitis/chronic pelvic pain syndrome: a meta-analysis of randomized controlled trials. J Androl 2006; 27(6):847–52.

[54] Mehik A, Alas P, Nickel JC, et al. Alfuzosin treatment for chronic prostatitis/chronic pelvic pain syndrome: a prospective, randomized, double-blind, placebo-controlled, pilot study. Urology 2003; 62(3):425–9.

[55] Cheah PY, Liong ML, Yuen KH, et al. Initial, long-term, and durable responses to terazosin, placebo, or other therapies for chronic prostatitis/chronic pelvic pain syndrome [see comment]. Urology 2004;64: 881–6.

[56] Nickel JC, Narayan P, McKay J, et al. Treatment of chronic prostatitis/chronic pelvic pain syndrome with tamsulosin: a randomized double blind trial. J Urol 2004;171:1594–7.

[57] Shoskes DA, Zeitlin SI, Shahed A, et al. Quercetin in men with category III chronic prostatitis: a preliminary prospective, double-blind, placebo-controlled trial. Urology 1999;54:960–3.

[58] Nickel JC, Forrest JB, Tomera K, et al. Pentosan polysulfate sodium therapy for men with chronic pelvic pain syndrome: a multicenter, randomized, placebo controlled study. J Urol 2005;173(4): 1252–5.

[59] Nickel JC, Barkin J, Forrest J, et al. Randomized, double-blind, dose-ranging study of pentosan polysulfate sodium for interstitial cystitis. Urology 2005;65:654–8.

[60] Nickel JC, Downey J, Pontari MA, et al. A randomized placebo-controlled multicentre study to evaluate the safety and efficacy of finasteride for male chronic pelvic pain syndrome (category IIIA chronic nonbacterial prostatitis) [see comment]. BJU Int 2004;93(7):991–5.

[61] Godfrey RG. A guide to the understanding and use of tricyclic antidepressants in the overall management of fibromyalgia and other chronic pain syndromes. Arch Intern Med 1996;156:1047–52. May 1027.

[62] Dworkin RH, Backonja M, Rowbotham MC, et al. Advances in neuropathic pain: diagnosis, mechanisms, and treatment recommendations [see comment]. Arch Neurol 2003;60:1524–34.

[63] Dworkin RH, Corbin AE, Young JP Jr, et al. Pregabalin for the treatment of postherpetic neuralgia: a randomized, placebo-controlled trial [see comment]. Neurology 2003;60(8):1274–83.

[64] Rosenstock J, Tuchman M, LaMoreaux L, et al. Pregabalin for the treatment of painful diabetic peripheral neuropathy: a double-blind, placebo-controlled trial. Pain 2004;110:628–38.

[65] Nickel JC. Opioids for chronic prostatitis and interstitial cystitis: lessons learned from the 11th World Congress on Pain. Urology 2006;68: 697–701.

[66] Anderson RU, Wise D, Sawyer T, et al. Integration of myofascial trigger point release and paradoxical relaxation training treatment of chronic pelvic pain in men [see comment]. J Urol 2005; 174(1):155–60.

[67] Anderson RU, Wise D, Sawyer T, et al. Sexual dysfunction in men with chronic prostatitis/chronic pelvic pain syndrome: improvement after trigger point release and paradoxical relaxation training. J Urol 2006;176(4 Pt 1):1534–8 [discussion: 1538–9].

[68] Chen R, Nickel JC. Acupuncture ameliorates symptoms in men with chronic prostatitis/chronic pelvic pain syndrome [see comment]. Urology 2003;61(6): 1156–9 [discussion: 1159].

[69] Zeitlin SI. Heat therapy in the treatment of prostatitis. Urology 2002;60(Suppl 6):38–40.

[70] Nickel JC, Downey J, Ardern D, et al. Failure of a monotherapy strategy for difficult chronic prostatitis/chronic pelvic pain syndrome [see comment]. J Urol 2004;172:551–4.

[71] Nickel JC, Berger RE, Pontari MA. Chronic pelvic pain—new pathways to discovery. Rev Urol 2006;8: 28–35.

ELSEVIER
SAUNDERS

Urol Clin N Am 35 (2008) 91–99

UROLOGIC
CLINICS
of North America

Re-imagining Interstitial Cystitis

Philip M. Hanno, MD, MPH

Hospital of the University of Pennsylvania, 9 Penn Tower, 3400 Spruce Street, Philadelphia, PA 19104, USA

New developments in infection/inflammation in urology Re-imagining interstitial cystitis

Since Keay [1] postulated an "antiproliferative factor" (APF) in 1998 and described this putative central protein in the etiologic pathway of the painful bladder syndrome/interstitial cystitis (PBS/IC) six years later [2], there have been no dramatic breakthroughs in the field. Although much potentially exciting work—largely funded by the National Institute of Diabetes, Digestive, and Kidney Disorders (NIDDK) and with the essential support of the Interstitial Cystitis Association (ICA)—is in progress with regard to epidemiology, etiology, and clinical treatment, many clinicians and researchers have used this hiatus to take another look at what exactly is being studied and how the syndrome should be approached. This article explores some of the current "hot-button" issues of definition and nomenclature that have formed the basis of many international meetings in the last 5 years.

Definition

"When I use a word," Humpty Dumpty said, in rather a scornful tone, "it means just what I choose it to mean—neither more nor less."
"The question is," said Alice, "whether you can make words mean so many different things."
"The question is," said Humpty Dumpty, "which is to be master—that's all." [3]

Tage Hald refered to it as "a hole in the air" [4]. It has been 20 years since the NIDDK proposed diagnostic criteria for entrance into research studies of interstitial cystitis (IC) [5,6], and so inadvertently defined the disorder for a generation of urologists. There has been a change in the way the disease (symptom complex, syndrome?) is perceived, and it is valuable to review briefly some of the ways it has been defined in the past (Box 1).

When the NIDDK-revised criteria were compared with the database entry criteria, it was apparent that up to 60% of patients clinically believed to have IC by experienced clinicians were being missed when the NIDDK research criteria were used as a definition of the disease (Fig. 1) [12].

The lack of clarity in terms of definition is highlighted when looking at the results of numerous epidemiology prevalence studies that show widely disparate results, depending on how the disorder is defined (Fig. 2) [13–18]. These studies show prevalence rates in 100,000 females, from 1.8 when physician-assigned diagnoses were used in Olmstead County, Minnesota, [19] to 450 when patients self-reported a diagnosis in the National Household Interview Survey [20]. Interestingly, rates are surprisingly similar in Finland, Taiwan, and Austria (at about 300) when a high O'Leary-Sant symptom score is used as a surrogate for a diagnosis of IC (see Fig. 2) [21–24].

Unfortunately, histopathology does not help when it comes to defining this symptom. One can have bladder biopsies consistent with the diagnosis of IC, but there is no microscopic picture pathognomonic of this disorder. The role of histopathology in the diagnosis of IC is primarily one of excluding other possible diagnoses. Rosamilia and colleagues reviewed the pathology literature pertaining to IC and presented their own data [25,26]. They compared forceps biopsies from 35 control and 34 IC patients, 6 with bladder capacities less than 400cc under anesthesia. Epithelial denudation, submucosal edema, congestion

E-mail address: hannop@uphs.upenn.edu

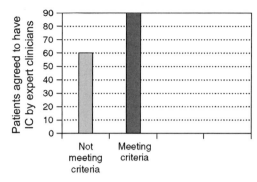

Fig. 1. NIDDK criteria compared with IC database entry criteria; 424 patients with urgency or pain or frequency greater than 6 months (see text for explanation). (*Data from* Hanno PM, Landis JR, Matthews-Cook Y, et al. The diagnosis of interstitial cystitis revisited: lessons learned from the National Institutes of Health Interstitial Cystitis Database study. J Urol 1999;161(2):553–7.)

findings, because transurethral resection biopsies tend to show mucosal ruptures, submucosal hemorrhage, and mild inflammation [27], whereas histology is normal approximately half the time with cold-cup forceps biopsies [28,29].

Keay's finding [30] that cells from the bladder lining of normal controls grow significantly more rapidly in culture than cells from IC patients, and her subsequent discovery and description of a frizzled 8 protein produced by bladder uroepithelial cells (APF) of IC patients, holds promise as a marker of the disease and, perhaps, a way to define it. As of 2007, neither have her findings been replicated by other centers, nor has a commercially available assay for APF been approved. The use of APF as a diagnostic marker and a part of the clinical definition of the syndrome remains tantalizing but not clinically accessible.

Is there a clinical test that, by virtue of its sensitivity and specificity, could be used to diagnose IC and thereby become a part of the definition of the disorder? Unfortunately, there is not. The potassium chloride test proposed by Parsons and colleagues [31]—an intravesical challenge comparing the sensory nerve provocative ability of saline versus potassium chloride using a 0.4M-KCl solution—has not gained acceptance as a diagnostic test for a variety of reasons [32]. It has neither the specificity nor the sensitivity to be used as a diagnostic test, and therefore results of the test could not be a part of any clinically useful definition.

As the new century dawned, there was much confusion as to how to define this 100-year-old

and ectasia, and inflammatory infiltrate were increased in the IC group. Submucosal hemorrhage did not differentiate the groups, but denuded epithelium was unique to the IC group and more common in those with severe disease. The most remarkable finding in this study was that histologic parameters were normal and indistinguishable from control subjects in 55% of IC patients. Method of biopsy can be important in interpreting

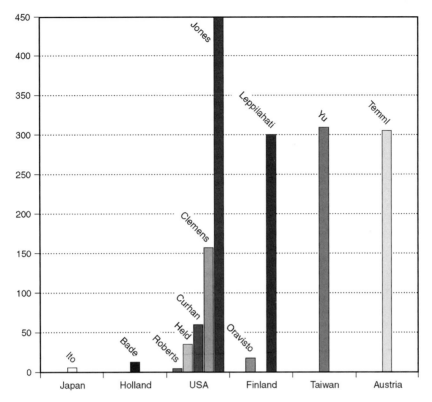

Fig. 2. IC prevalence per 100,000 female population (see text for explanation).

syndrome, and the need for a clinically useful, universally accepted way to characterize IC took to the forefront. Abrams and the International Continence Society (ICS) preferred Bourke's term "painful bladder" and defined painful bladder syndrome as "the complaint of suprapubic pain related to bladder filling, accompanied by other symptoms such as increased daytime and night-time frequency, in the absence of proven urinary infection or other obvious pathology." Rather than drop the designation of IC all together, they limited it to patients with painful bladder who had "typical cystoscopic and histological features" without identifying those features [33]. The term "urgency" was effectively taken out of the IC equation, and used to identify "*the complaint of a sudden compelling desire to pass urine which is difficult to defer.*" It became an integral part of the definition of overactive bladder: *urgency with or without urge incontinence, usually with frequency and nocturia.* Some degree of confusion has resulted [34], and patient organizations have not been happy to give up the urgency term, one that many patients identify with their IC

symptoms [35]. When looking at the Interstitial Cystitis Symptom Index (O'Leary-Sant ICSI), the ICSI question for urgency, "the strong need to urinate with little or no warning," consistently yields lower scores than the severity question of "the compelling urge to urinate that is difficult to postpone" [36].

Warren [37] compared the ICS painful bladder criteria with symptoms of patients he recruited for a case control study of newly diagnosed women with IC. His criteria for entrance into the study included women greater than 18 years of age with symptom onset within 12 months. They had greater than 4 weeks of perceived bladder pain at or greater than 3 on a 10-point Likert scale and at least two of frequency ($\geq 8/24$ hours), urgency (≥ 3 on a Likert scale), or nocturia. Exclusionary criteria were those of the NIDDK. He found that the ICS definition identified only 66% of his 138 cases. Those who met the definition did not differ from those who did not. The restriction to "suprapubic pain" in the ICS definition and the relationship of pain to filling were the criteria most responsible for the poor sensitivity.

Soon after the ICS terminology publication, several high-profile international meetings were held to tackle the problem of definition and nomenclature and establish a new framework for future collaborative research. Although each meeting had long, complex agendas, it is useful to look at how each approached the definition of the syndrome.

The first of these meetings was the International Consultation on Interstitial Cystitis Japan (ICICJ), held in Kyoto in March 2003, under the direction of Ueda, Sant, Yoshimura, and the present author [38]. This meeting concluded by suggesting the following:

Interstitial cystitis should be suspected and further investigation is recommended in any patients with pelvic pain and urgency and/or urinary frequency associated with no obvious treatable condition/ pathology. The term IC should be expanded to a term IC/CPPS (interstitial cystitis/chronic pelvic pain syndrome) when pelvic pain is at least of 3 months duration and associated with no obvious treatable condition/pathology.

The ICICJ was quickly followed by a meeting of a newly formed European Society for the Study of IC (ESSIC). The first meeting was held in Denmark in May 2003, with annual meetings thereafter. A process was begun that culminated in 2005 with the acceptance by ESSIC of the ICS definition of PBS with only minor modification [39]. IC was a subset of PBS defined as:

A disease of unknown origin consisting of the complaint of suprapubic pain related to bladder filling accompanied by other symptoms, such as increased daytime ($>8\times$) and nighttime ($>1\times$) frequency, and with cystoscopic (glomerulations and/or Hunner's lesions) and/or histological features (mononuclear inflammatory cells including mast cell infiltration and granulation tissue) in the absence of infection or other pathology.

On October 29 2003, the NIDDK convened a meeting of the members of the Interstitial Cystitis Epidemiology Task Force, the IC executive committee, ad hoc participants, and National Institutes of Health staff to review the status of current investigations of IC and to plan new epidemiology investigations [40]. The following served as their working definition:

Interstitial cystitis is a symptomatic diagnosis based on the presence of three key symptoms: pain, urgency, and frequency, as well as exclusion of a short list of other conditions that cause the same symptoms. Pain is the most consistent and

disabling symptom for IC patients. Some will not use the term pain, but will rather describe a sense of pressure or discomfort. Typically, but not always, the pain is worse with filling of the bladder and is relieved by emptying of the bladder. Urgency in IC patients differs from that experienced by patients with urinary incontinence. In IC patients, the urgency is driven by pain, in patients with incontinence (detrusor overactivity), it is driven by their fear of losing control. Not enough information is available on normal variability of urinary frequency to establish a number that can help diagnose IC.

Immediately following the epidemiology meeting, the NIDDK, in conjunction with the ICA, held a basic and clinical science symposium [41]. It concluded: "The struggle to define IC will continue. Bladder pain will continue to be the key to the definition in the near future."

In June 2004 the third International Consultation on Incontinence, cosponsored by the International Consultation on Urological Diseases in official relationship with the World Health Organization, the International Society of Urology, the ICS, and the major international associations of Urology and Gynecology, adopted the ICS definition of IC and PBS. It noted that because of the ambiguity in defining IC as a subset of PBS, the terms would be used together to refer to the same constellation of symptoms (PBS/IC) [25]. Further, it concluded that: "Interstitial cystitis is a clinical diagnosis primarily based on symptoms of urgency/frequency and pain in the bladder and or pelvis. The combined term PBS/ IC will be used until more specific criteria can be established."

Soon after the International Consultation on Incontinence, the Multinational Interstitial Cystitis Association met to carry the discussion forward [41]. The group kept the ICS definition of PBS, but broadened the symptom of pain to include "pressure" and "discomfort." The group went on to note:

Interstitial cystitis may be a subgroup of this larger syndrome (PBS) ... but as this remains somewhat vague, a general nomenclature is preferred and the question of what is "IC" alone is left to be determined. Urgency is a common complaint of this group of patients. The ICS definition of urgency could be interpreted as compatible with either detrusor overactivity of PBS/IC. Because the term of urgency would tend to obfuscate the borders of these two conditions and may be unnecessary as a part of the definition of PBS/IC, its place in the definition will need to be worked out in conjunction with the ICS terminology committee.

The ESSIC presented a comprehensive report at the NIDDK 2006 "Frontiers in Painful Bladder Syndrome and Interstitial Cystitis" meeting in October 2006. In response to a decision made public there by the ESSIC to drop the moniker "interstitial cystitis" in favor of "bladder pain syndrome"—which was to be further categorized by results of optional investigations (see below)—the ICA, in conjunction with the Association of Reproductive Health Professionals, held a meeting in Washington, DC. The meeting included a cross-section of invited American urologists, gynecologists, nurses, and representatives from the German patient organization and a urologist from Germany. The following definition was promulgated at the meeting and is available at http://www.arhp.org/healthcareproviders/visiting facultyprograms/icpbs/whitepaper.cfm: IC/PBS is defined by pelvic pain, pressure, or discomfort related to the bladder, typically associated with persistent urge to void or urinary frequency, in the absence of infection or other pathology.

The term "persistent urge" was meant to include the idea of urgency in the definition while not directly impinging on the ICS's use of the term as defined for overactive bladder.

In a compromise presented at the second International Consultation on Interstitial Cystitis Japan, in March 2007, the ESSIC agreed to modify the name and definition to be acceptable to all stakeholders. This was confirmed at their meeting in Muenster, in May 2007.

> Bladder pain syndrome/interstitial cystitis would be diagnosed on the basis of chronic pelvic pain, pressure or discomfort perceived to be related to the urinary bladder accompanied by at least one other urinary symptoms like persistent urge to void or urinary frequency. Confusable diseases as the cause of the symptoms must be excluded.
>
> Further documentation and classification of BPB/IC might be performed according to findings at cystoscopy with hydrodistention and morphological findings in bladder biopsies.

Nomenclature

Following closely on the heals of definition is nomenclature. In many ways this has morphed in to a hot-button issue, and in mid-2007 there is no agreement as to how this complex syndrome should be referred to.

Changes in nomenclature have punctuated the literature over the last 170 years. The syndrome has variously been referred to as tic douloureux of the bladder, IC, cystitis parenchymatosa, Hunner's ulcer, panmural ulcerative cystitis, urethral syndrome, and PBS [7,9,42–46]. The term "interstitial cystitis," which Skene is credited with coining and Hunner for bringing it in to common usage, is somewhat of a misnomer; in many cases not only is there no interstitial inflammation, but also, histopathologically, there may be no inflammation at all [26,28,47,48].

With the formal definition of the term "painful bladder syndrome" by the ICS in 2002 [33], the terminology discussion began to take on an importance and priority not seen for decades. Perhaps the lack of progress in identifying causes of the disorder and effective treatments might somehow be related to an improper focus solely on bladder pathology, partly as a result of the potentially misleading name of the disorder. Was the perspective of researchers and clinicians somehow off target, and should this disorder be looked at as part of a new paradigm (perhaps through a pain paradigm)?

In Kyoto at the ICICJ in March 2003, it was agreed that the term "interstitial cystitis" should be expanded to "interstitial cystitis/chronic pelvic pain syndrome" when pelvic pain is at least of 3 months duration and associated with no obvious treatable condition/pathology [38]. The ESSIC held its first meeting in Copenhagen soon after Kyoto. Nomenclature was discussed, but no decision was reached, as the meeting concentrated on how to evaluate patients for diagnosis [49]. At the 2003 meeting of the NIDDK titled, "Research Insights into Interstitial Cystitis," it was concluded that "interstitial cystitis" will inexorably be replaced as a *sole* name for this syndrome. It will be a gradual process over several years. At the meeting it was referred to as "interstitial cystitis/painful bladder syndrome" in keeping with ICS nomenclature [41].

At the 2004 meeting of the Multinational Interstitial Cystitis Association in Rome, it was concluded that the syndrome should be referred to as "painful bladder syndrome/interstitial cystitis" or "PBS/IC" [41]. That same year, the International Consultation on Incontinence, cosponsored by the ICS and Societe Internationale d''Urologie in association with the World Health Organization, included the syndrome as a part of the consultation. Interestingly, the chapter in the report was titled, "painful bladder syndrome (including interstitial cystitis)," suggesting that the IC formed an identifiable subset within the broader syndrome. Because such a distinction is difficult to define, within the body of the chapter, co-authored by nine committee members and five consultants from four continents, it was referred to as PBS/IC (one inclusive entity) [25].

In June 2006 Abrams and colleagues [50] published an editorial that attacked the nomenclature problem head-on. They noted that:

> It is an advantage if the medical term has clear diagnostic features that translate to a known pathophysiologic process so that effective treatment may be given. Unfortunately, the latter is not the case for many of the pain syndromes suffered by patients seen at most pain, gynecological, and urological clinics. For the most part these "diagnoses" describe syndromes that do not have recognized standard definitions, yet infer knowledge of a pathophysiologic cause for the symptoms. Unfortunately the terminology used to describe the condition may promote erroneous thinking about treatment on the part of physicians, surgeons and patients. These organ based diagnoses are mysterious, misleading and unhelpful, and can lead to therapies that are misguided or even dangerous.

The editorial went on to note that a single pathologic descriptive term (interstitial cystitis) for a spectrum of symptom combinations ill serves patients. The umbrella term "painful bladder syndrome" was proposed, with a goal to define and investigate subsets of patients who could be clearly identified within the spectrum of PBS. It would fall within the rubric of chronic pelvic pain syndrome. Sufferers would be identified according to the primary organ that *appears* to be affected on clinical grounds. Pain not associated with an individual organ would be described in terms of the symptoms. One can see in this the beginnings of a new paradigm that might be expected to change the emphasis of both clinical and basic science research, and that removes the automatic presumption that the end-organ in the name of the disease should necessarily be the sole or primary target of such research.

At the major biannual IC research conference in the fall of 2006, held by the NIDDK (Frontiers in Painful Bladder Syndrome—PBS and Interstitial Cystitis), the ESSIC group was given a block of time with which to present their thoughts and conclusions [51]. Because PBS did not fit into the taxonomy of other pelvic pain syndromes such as urethral or vulvar pain syndromes, and because

IC is open to different interpretations, ESSIC decided to rename PBS as bladder pain syndrome (BPS), followed by a type designation. BPS is indicated by two symbols, the first of which corresponds to cystoscopy with hydrodistention findings (1, 2, or 3, indicating increasing grade of severity) and the second to biopsy (A, B, and C, indicating increasing grade of severity of biopsy findings). Although neither cystoscopy with hydrodistention nor bladder biopsy was prescribed as an essential part of the evaluation, by categorizing patients as to whether either procedure was done, and if so, the results, it is possible to follow patients with similar findings and study each identified cohort to compare natural history, prognosis, and response to therapy.

Table 1 shows the layout of this type of classification with notation as to what previously was termed "PBS" and what would fall into past definitions of IC. Both terms become superfluous for purposes of categorization if one adopts the ESSIC classification of BPS with the appropriate letter and number. As Baranowski [52] conceives it, BPS is thus defined as pain with a collection of symptoms, the most important of which is pain perceived to be in the bladder. IC is distinguished as an end-organ, visceral-neural pain syndrome, whereas BPS can be considered a pain syndrome that involves the end-organ (bladder) and neuro-visceral (myopathic) mechanisms. In IC, one expects end-organ primary pathology. This is not necessarily the case in the broader BPS (Table 1).

Another way to conceptualize this is with the drawing of a target (Fig. 3).

There may be many causes of chronic pelvic pain. When an etiology cannot be determined, it is characterized as pelvic pain syndrome. To the extent that it can be distinguished as urologic, gynecologic, dermatologic, and the like, it is further categorized by organ system. A urologic pain syndrome can sometimes be further differentiated on the site of perceived pain. Bladder, prostate, testicular, and epididymal pain syndromes follow. Finally, types of BPS can be further defined as IC, or simply categorized by ESSIC criteria. This new perspective, which remains in its formative stages, will likely be presented in a more crystallized form by Andrew Baranowski as a part of the International Association for the Study of Pain Conference, in Glasgow in 2008.

Patient groups have expressed significant reservations with regard to any nomenclature change

Table 1
Classification of bladder pain syndrome by the European Society for the study of Interstitial Cystitis (see text for explanation)

ESSIC Classification of BPS

CYSTOSCOPY WITH HYDRODISTENTION

		Not Done	Normal	Glomerulations	Hunner Lesion
BIOPSY	Not Done	XX PBS	1X PBS	2X IC	3X IC
	Normal	XA PBS	1A PBS	2A IC	3A IC
	Inconclusive	XB PBS	1B PBS	2B IC	3B IC
	Positive	XC IC	1C IC	2C IC	3C IC

Nordling J and van de Merwe JP. ESSIC web site, Accessed, September 2006.

(*Data from* Nordling J. ESSIC classification of BPS/IC. European Opinion on PBS/IC Characterizations. Presented at the 2006 International Symposium Frontiers in Painful Bladder Syndrome and Interstitial Cystitis, National Institute of Diabetes and Digestive and Kidney Disease. Bethesda, MD, October 26–27, 2006.)

that potentially drops the "interstitial cystitis" moniker. The meeting organized by the Association of Reproductive Health Professionals and the ICA concluded that:

> The nomenclature of IC/PBS may need to change, but change should not be undertaken now because there is insufficient evidence to support a change. Any change in nomenclature

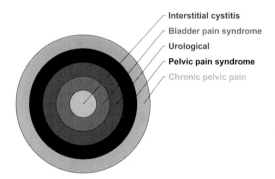

Fig. 3. Proposed classification system for chronic pain syndromes, where IC might fit in (initial proposal by Baronowski [51]). (*Data from* Nordling J. ESSIC classification of BPS/IC. European Opinion on PBS/IC Characterizations. Presented at the 2006 International Symposium Frontiers in Painful Bladder Syndrome and Interstitial Cystitis, National Institute of Diabetes and Digestive and Kidney Disease. Bethesda, MD, October 26–27, 2006.)

should be evidence-based. This group favors retaining IC in whatever name is considered in the future and positioning it first, as in IC/PBS [35].

Their objections include the following:

1. BPS is too broad a term
2. Name change will result in decreased recognition of the syndrome after years of efforts to increase awareness of the name IC
3. Patients, legislators, and the general public will be adversely impacted by a name change
4. The U.S. Social Security Administration and private insurance recognizes IC but not the term BPS, and benefits could be adversely affected
5. A negative impact on research funding is possible
6. A negative impact on literature searches and information gathering is possible

As a result of these concerns, the ESSIC plans to append the IC term to the BPS nomenclature for the foreseeable future, referring to the syndrome as BPS/IC.

Next steps

The worldwide community of health care professionals rely on the use of a single medical language to communicate. Ideally, terminology should be easily recognizable throughout the global medical community. Although much of the discussion may seem pedantic, it is in reality of the utmost importance and represents nothing short of a new paradigm with which to view the IC syndrome in a new context. Efforts to establish a consensus for a clinical definition, nomenclature, and diagnostic algorithm through the auspices of the American Urological Association and the European Association of Urology are underway. The NIDDK is planning similar meetings to bring together a definition and appropriate nomenclature for the clinical and basic research community. It is hoped that these efforts will be somehow linked to provide a conclusion satisfactory to all stakeholders, and which is consistent worldwide. Hopefully, the U.S. Food and Drug Administration will find the efforts worthwhile, and signal the pharmaceutical industry how best to proceed with clinical research studies based on the paradigm so that the field can advance for the benefit of all patients.

References

[1] Keay S, Warren JW. A hypothesis for the etiology of interstitial cystitis based upon inhibition of bladder epithelial repair. Med Hypotheses 1998;51(1): 79–83.

[2] Keay SK, Szekely Z, Conrads TP, et al. An antiproliferative factor from interstitial cystitis patients is a frizzled 8 protein-related sialoglycopeptide. Proc Natl Acad Sci USA 2004;101(32):11803–8.

[3] Carroll L. Humpty dumpty. Through the looking glass. Public Domain; 1871.

[4] George NJR. Preface. In: George NJR, Gosling JA, editors. Sensory disorders of the bladder and urethra. Berlin: Springer-Verlag; 1986. p. vii.

[5] Gillenwater JY, Wein AJ. Summary of the national institute of arthritis, diabetes, digestive and kidney diseases workshop on interstitial cystitis, National Institutes of Health, Bethesda, Maryland, August 28–29, 1987. J Urol 1988;140(1):203–6.

[6] Wein A, Hanno PM, Gillenwater JY. Interstitial cystitis: an introduction to the problem. In: Hanno PM, Staskin DR, Krane RJ, et al, editors. Interstitial cystitis. London: Springer-Verlag; 1990. p. 3–15.

[7] Skene AJC. Diseases of the bladder and urethra in women. New York: William Wood; 1887.

[8] Hunner GL. A rare type of bladder ulcer in women; report of cases. Boston Med Surg Journal 1915;172: 660–4.

[9] Bourque JP. Surgical management of the painful bladder. J Urol 1951;65:25–34.

[10] Messing EM, Stamey TA. Interstitial cystitis: early diagnosis, pathology, and treatment. Urology 1978;12(4):381–92.

[11] Simon LJ, Landis JR, Tomaszewski JE, et al. The interstitial cystitis database (ICDB) study. In: Sant GR, editor. Interstitial cystitis. Philadelphia: Lippincott-Raven; 1997. p. 17–24.

[12] Hanno PM, Landis JR, Matthews-Cook Y, et al. The diagnosis of interstitial cystitis revisited: lessons learned from the National Institutes of Health Interstitial Cystitis Database study. J Urol 1999;161(2): 553–7.

[13] Oravisto KJ. Epidemiology of interstitial cystitis. Ann Chir Gynaecol Fenn 1975;64(2):75–7.

[14] Ito T, Miki M, Yamada T. Interstitial cystitis in Japan. BJU Int 2000;86(6):634–7.

[15] Held PJ, Hanno PM, Wein AJ. Epidemiology of interstitial cystitis: 2. In: Hanno PM, Staskin DR, Krane RJ, et al, editors. Interstitial cystitis. London: Springer-Verlag; 1990. p. 29–48.

[16] Curhan GC, Speizer FE, Hunter DJ, et al. Epidemiology of interstitial cystitis: a population based study. J Urol 1999;161(2):549–52.

[17] Clemens J, Meenan R, Rosetti M, et al. Prevalence and incidence of interstitial cystitis in a managed care population. J Urol 2005;173:98–102.

[18] Bade JJ, Rijcken B, Mensink HJ. Interstitial cystitis in The Netherlands: prevalence, diagnostic criteria and therapeutic preferences. J Urol 1995;154(6): 2035–7.

[19] Roberts RO, Bergstralh EJ, Bass SE, et al. Incidence of physician-diagnosed interstitial cystitis in Olmsted County: a community-based study. BJU Int 2003;91(3):181–5.

[20] Jones CA, Nyberg L. Prevalence of interstitial cystitis in the United States [Abstract]. J Urol 1994;151: 423A.

[21] Yu H-J. Prevalence of interstitial cystitis in Taiwan. Presented at Pan Asian Interstitial Cystitis Conference, Tapei, Taiwan, April 2006.

[22] Temml C, Wehrberger C, Riedl C, et al. Prevalence and correlates for interstitial cystitis symptoms in women participating in a health screening project. Eur Urol 2007;51(3):803–8.

[23] Leppilahti M, Tammela TL, Huhtala H, et al. Prevalence of symptoms related to interstitial cystitis in women: a population based study in Finland. J Urol 2002;168(1):139–43.

[24] Leppilahti M, Sairanen J, Tammela TL, et al. Prevalence of clinically confirmed interstitial cystitis in women: a population based study in Finland. J Urol 2005;174(2):581–3.

[25] Hanno P, Baranowski A, Fall M, et al. Painful bladder syndrome (including interstitial cystitis). In: Abrams PH, Wein AJ, Cardozo L, editors. Incontinence. 3rd edition. Paris: Health Publications Limited; 2005. p. 1456–520.

[26] Rosamilia A, Igawa Y, Higashi S. Pathology of interstitial cystitis. Int J Urol 2003;10 Suppl:S11–5.

[27] Johansson SL, Fall M. Clinical features and spectrum of light microscopic changes in interstitial cystitis. J Urol 1990;143(6):1118–24.

[28] Lynes WL, Flynn SD, Shortliffe LD, et al. The histology of interstitial cystitis. Am J Surg Pathol 1990;14(10):969–76.

[29] Mattila J. Vascular immunopathology in interstitial cystitis. Clin Immunol Immunopathol 1982;23(3):648–55.

[30] Keay S, Zhang CO, Marvel R, et al. Antiproliferative factor, heparin-binding epidermal growth factor-like growth factor, and epidermal growth factor: sensitive and specific urine markers for interstitial cystitis. Urology 2001;57(6 Suppl 1):104–7.

[31] Parsons CL, Greenberger M, Gabal L, et al. The role of urinary potassium in the pathogenesis and diagnosis of interstitial cystitis. J Urol 1998;159(6):1862–6.

[32] Hanno P. Is the potassium sensitivity test a valid and useful test for the diagnosis of interstitial cystitis? Int Urogynecol J Pelvic Floor Dysfunct 2005;16(6):428–9.

[33] Abrams PH, Cardozo L, Fall M, et al. The standardisation of terminology of lower urinary tract function: report from the standardisation sub-committee of the international continence society. Neurourology and Urodynamics 2002;21:167–78.

[34] Abrams P, Hanno P, Wein A. Overactive bladder and painful bladder syndrome: there need not be confusion. Neurourol Urodyn 2005;24(2):149–50.

[35] Outcome of the Washington, DC, Consensus Meeting on Interstitial Cystitis/Painful Bladder Syndrome: Association of Reproductive Health Professionals; 2007.

[36] Diggs C, Meyer WA, Langenberg P, et al. Assessing urgency in interstitial cystitis/painful bladder syndrome. Urology 2007;69(2):210–4.

[37] Warren JW, Meyer WA, Greenberg P, et al. Using the International Continence Society's definition of painful bladder syndrome. Urology 2006;67(6):1138–42.

[38] Ueda T, Sant G, Hanno P, et al. International Consultation on Interstitial Cystitis Japan. International Journal of Urology 2003;10(Supplement):1–70.

[39] Van De Merwe J, Nordling J. Interstitial cystitis: definitions and confusable diseases; ESSIC meeting 2005 Baden. European Urology Today [March 2006], 14–17, 2006.

[40] Vaughn ED, Wilt T, Hanno P, et al. Epidemiology of interstitial cystitis, executive committee summary and task force report. 2004 Oct 29; Two Democracy Plaza, 7'th Floor. Bethesda (MD): National Institutes of Health; 2003.

[41] Hanno P, Keay S, Moldwin R, et al. International Consultation on IC—Rome, September 2004. Forging an International Consensus: progress in painful bladder syndrome/interstitial cystitis. Report and abstracts. Int Urogynecol J Pelvic Floor Dysfunct 2005;16(Suppl 1):S2–34.

[42] Christmas TJ. Historical aspects of interstitial cystitis. In: Sant GR, editor. Interstitial cystitis. Philadelphia: Lippincott-Raven; 1997. p. 1–8.

[43] Hunner GL. A rare type of bladder ulcer. Further notes, with a report of eighteen cases. JAMA 1918;70(4):203–12.

[44] Parsons JK, Parsons CL. The historical origins of interstitial cystitis. J Urol 2004;171(1):20–2.

[45] Powell NB, Powell EB. The female urethra: a clinicopathological study. J Urol 1949;61:557–70.

[46] Teichman JM, Thompson IM, Taichman NS. Joseph Parrish, tic doloureux of the bladder and interstitial cystitis. J Urol 2000;164(5):1473–5.

[47] Denson MA, Griebling TL, Cohen MB, et al. Comparison of cystoscopic and histological findings in patients with suspected interstitial cystitis. J Urol 2000;164(6):1908–11.

[48] Tomaszewski JE, Landis JR, Russack V, et al. Biopsy features are associated with primary symptoms in interstitial cystitis: results from the interstitial cystitis database study. Urology 2001;57(6 Suppl 1):67–81.

[49] Nordling J. Overview of the European Copenhagen workshop on interstitial cystitis, Denmark—May 2003. Int Urogynecol 2005;16(S):14–5.

[50] Abrams P, Baranowski A, Berger R, et al. A new classification is needed for pelvic pain syndromes—are existing terminologies of spurious diagnostic authority bad for patients? J Urol 2006;175:1989–90.

[51] NIDDK. Frontiers in Painful Bladder Syndrome and Interstitial Cystitis, 2006. Available at: http://www3.niddk.nih.gov/fund/other/niddkfrontiers/. Accessed October 13, 2007.

[52] Baranowski AP, et al. Diagnostic criteria, classification, and nomenclature for painful bladder syndrome/interstitial cystitis: an essic proposal. European Urology 2007. doi:10.1016/j.eururo.2007.10.010.

ELSEVIER
SAUNDERS

Urol Clin N Am 35 (2008) 101–108

UROLOGIC
CLINICS
of North America

Diagnosis and Management of Epididymitis

Chad R. Tracy, MD*, William D. Steers, MD[1],
Raymond Costabile, MD[2]

*Department of Urology, University of Virginia School of Medicine, 1335 Lee Street, Charlottesville,
VA 22908, USA*

A variety of inflammatory conditions target the epididymis, including bacterial, viral, and fungal infections as well as idiopathic inflammation. Acute epididymitis is characterized by inflammation of the epididymis presenting as pain and swelling, generally occurring on one side and developing over several days. Multiple objective findings of epididymitis have been identified and, in variable degrees, may include positive urine cultures, fever, erythema of the scrotal skin, leukocytosis, urethritis, hydrocele, and involvement of the adjacent testis.

The true prevalence of epididymitis is unknown. Although epididymitis has been reported at any time from infancy up to 90 years of age, it is the fifth most common urologic diagnosis in men between the ages of 18 and 50 [1], with a mean patient age at presentation of 41 years [2]. The majority of patients are 20 to 39 years old (43%), followed by those 40 to 59 years old (29%) [2]. Of men presenting to Canadian outpatient urologists, 1% are diagnosed with epididymitis, with 80% of these patients having chronic epididymitis (>3 months) [3]. Although the financial impact of epididymitis on the health system is unknown, the morbidity of epididymitis is significant, with epididymitis accounting for a greater loss of man-hours in the United States military than any other urologic diagnosis [4].

The pathophysiology of acute epididymitis remains unclear, although it is postulated to occur

secondary to retrograde flow of infected urine into the ejaculatory duct. This hypothesis is strengthened by the finding that 56% of men older than 60 with epididymitis exhibit lower urinary tract obstruction, including benign prostatic hyperplasia, prostate cancer, and urethral stricture at the time of diagnosis [5]. In addition, multiple animal models have shown that injection of *Escherichia coli* or *Chlamydia trachomatis* into the vas deferens results in epididymitis that mimics clinical and microbiological findings of human epididymitis [6–8]. Control populations in these animal trials failed to develop epididymitis with injection of transport medium, though no studies have attempted injection of sterile urine into the vas deferens.

Infectious epididymitis

Evidence supporting retrograde inoculation of the epididymis from infected urine is supported by the increased risk of epididymitis following instrumentation of the urethra or bladder. In particular, patients who have infected urine during instrumentation are at highest risk for infectious epididymitis. Patients with complicated urinary tract infections, such as those requiring clean intermittent catheterization, account for 50% of all patients with infectious epididymitis [2,8,9]. Up to 80% of all cases of epididymitis may be bacterial in origin [10–13], though large epidemiologic studies have identified a clear bacterial etiology in fewer than 25% of subjects with clinical signs of epididymitis [2,9]. Transmission of *C trachomatis* is felt to be responsible for infectious epididymitis in patients 35 years old or younger, though the majority of men in this age range with epididymitis (up to 90%) have no objective

* Corresponding author.
E-mail address: ct5t@virginia.edu (C.R. Tracy).
[1] Consultant/investigator for Pfizer, Astellis, Sanofi-Aventis, Lilly.
[2] Consultant/investigator for Boehringer Ingelheim, Allergan, and Lilly Icos.

laboratory evidence of *C trachomatis* on urethral swab polymerase chain reaction [10,14–16]. In patients older than 35, coliform bacteria are the most common pathogens isolated in infectious epididymitis, with *E coli* accounting for the majority of cases. Other reports have sporadically implicated other bacteria that may be found in epididymitis, including *Ureaplasma urealyticum*, *Corynebacterium sp*, *Mycoplasma sp*, and *Mima polymorph* [17].

Clinical epididymitis in children identified through ultrasonography or surgical exploration has often been attributed to viral infections. A prospective study by Somekh and colleagues [18], using viral cultures of throat, urine, and stool specimens and serologic tests for common viruses, revealed significantly elevated titers to certain pathogens in patients with epididymitis compared with controls, including *M pneumoniae* (53% versus 20%), enteroviruses (62.5% versus 10%), and adenoviruses (20% versus 0%). Mumps infection, which was a frequent cause of viral epididymoorchitis in the past, has been virtually eliminated since the introduction of mumps vaccine in the United States in 1985. Because the majority of pediatric epididymitis is thought to be due to a viral etiology, management of nonbacterial epididymitis in children, defined by absence of pyuria, is often treated conservatively with ice and analgesics [19], which is in stark contrast to treatment of the adult population [2].

Chronic infectious epididymitis is most frequently seen in conditions associated with granulomatous reaction [20], with *Mycobacterium tuberculosis* (TB) being the most common granulomatous disease affecting the epididymis. Although renal involvement is often seen with epididymal TB, seeding of the epididymis is thought to occur from hematogenous spread of *M tuberculosis* rather than seeding of the urinary system via the kidneys [21]. Up to 25% of patients may have bilateral disease, with ultrasound demonstrating an enlarged hyperemic epididymis with multiple cysts and calcifications. Tuberculous epididymitis should be suspected in all patients with a known history of or recent exposure to TB, or in patients whose clinical status worsens despite appropriate antibiotic treatment. In addition, urologists must be cognizant of epididymoorchitis related to Bacille Calmette-Guérin, which may occur following treatment of superficial bladder cancer [22].

Genito-urinary TB is often difficult to diagnose as organisms are identified in the urine in less than half of the cases [23] and tuberculin skin testing is not specific for epididymal involvement. When present, cultures of a draining scrotal sinus may be used to identify epididymal TB. If a patient without a history of TB is confirmed to have tuberculous epididymitis, he should undergo the appropriate evaluation for systemic TB, including chest X ray, renal function tests, and CT or excretory urography if indicated.

Brucella is a gram-negative facultative coccobacillus that causes epididymitis in up to 10% of patients with brucellosis [24]. Infection with *Brucella* typically occurs from direct contact with infected animals or ingestion of their nonpasteurized milk, and primarily occurs in endemic areas [25]. In the United States brucellosis occurs primarily in California and Texas owing to their proximity to the Mexican border [25]. Patients with *Brucella* epididymitis are clinically similar to those with other causes of infectious epididymitis, although they are more likely to have complex septated hydroceles on ultrasound examination [26]. The diagnosis of brucellosis can be confirmed based on patient history and serologic testing that demonstrates a single titer of above 1:160 or a greater than fourfold increase in agglutinating antibodies during a 4- to 12-week period.

Although rare in the United States, funiculoepididymitis may occur from filarial invasion of the lymphatic system, leading to scarring and formation of cord masses, large hydroceles, and lymphedema [27]. More than 90% of human lymphatic filariasis are caused by *Wucheria bancrofti*, with *Brugia timori* and *B malayi* accounting for the remainder of cases. Infection typically centers in the epididymis and lower spermatic cord, and then spreads centrifugally. Death of the microfilaria leads to development of fever, localized lymphangitis, edema, and hydrocele. In addition, patients may present with chyluria owing to lymphatic obstruction. Ultrasound typically reveals enlarged lymphatic channels, and real-time imaging may demonstrate random movements of viable microfilaria ("dance sign"). Definitive diagnosis relies on identification of filaria on peripheral blood smear.

Noninfectious epididymitis

Although it is recognized that a large number of patients with epididymal inflammation have no evidence of genitourinary infection, little direct evidence is available regarding the mechanism of noninfectious epididymitis. One proposed mechanism is the retrograde reflux of sterile urine into the vas deferens from contraction of a full bladder against a closed external urethral sphincter. However, multiple reviews attempting to confirm this concept have identified fewer than 10% of patients with a documented history of straining to void [2,9,10]. Although the reflux of sterile urine into the vas deferens may occur when men with nonobstructed bladder outlets or urethras strain to void, little evidence is available to support this mechanism as having a primary role in noninfectious epididymitis. In addition, the present authors' own experience reveals that men who have undergone vasectomy can present years later with noninfectious clinical testis or epididymal swelling and pain, possibly arguing against retrograde inoculation of the epididymis as the sole contributor to epididymitis. Postvasectomy epididymal enlargement or pain has been attributed to congestion and inflammation owing to obstruction or sperm granuloma formation, which causes local reaction surrounding nerves and vasculature [28].

Sarcoidosis, a noninfectious, noncaseating, chronic granulomatous disease that is more common in black patients, affects the genitourinary system in up to 5% of cases [20,29]. Genitourinary manifestations include nephrocalcinosis; uremia; and granulomas of the epididymis, testis, and vas deferens, as well as cutaneous genital lesions. The typical presentation involves progressive enlargement of the epididymis in patients with a known history of sarcoidosis, occurring bilaterally in up to 30% of patients [29]. Ultrasound findings are variable, but often reveal an enlarged heterogeneous epididymis that may contain distinct nodules [30–32]. Treatment with corticosteroids relieves pain and swelling in the majority of cases and should be used before consideration of scrotal exploration. In the rare patient requiring exploration, frozen sectioning should be performed to prevent needless epididymectomy or orchiectomy [29]. In addition, patients should be counseled preoperatively on the risks of testicular damage with epididymal exploration.

Sarcoid involvement of the epididymis can lead to azoospermia owing to extrinsic compression of epididymal ducts, so semen analysis should be obtained at disease diagnosis in all patients interested in paternity and those undergoing scrotal exploration [33]. If oligospermia is noted, the patient should be offered the use of sperm banking for possible future assisted reproductive techniques. Steroid therapy may assist with transient restoration of genital tract patency and use; serial semen analysis may be useful for detecting rare sperm that may be banked in patients with azoospermia [34].

Several cases of noninfectious epididymitis have been linked to Behçet's disease—an idiopathic, multiorgan vasculitic disease displaying a large number of signs and symptoms, including recurrent aphthous ulcers, genital ulcers, uveitis, and epididymitis. Genital ulcers, which are tender to touch, are most common on the scrotum, although they may occur on the prepuce, glans, or penile shaft. To date, there have been no reports of patients with Behçet's presenting with objective evidence of urethritis or infection on urinalysis, urethral swab, or urine culture. Patients with epididymal involvement are more likely to have genital ulcers, cutaneous involvement, and arthritis than those without epididymal involvement [35]. Medical therapy for Behçet's disease is limited, with treatment primarily revolving around symptomatic relief and empiric treatment with topical or systemic corticosteroids.

Epididymitis can also be caused by medications, most notably the anti-arrhythmic amiodarone HCl [36]. High levels of this drug are achieved in the epididymis relative to serum (300 ×), leading to development of anti-amiodarone HCl antibodies that then attack the epididymis lining, resulting in pain and swelling. The incidence of epididymitis appears to be dose related, with clinical epididymitis developing in up to 11% of patients on high-dose amiodarone HCl [37]. Temporary discontinuation of the drug or a decrease in dosage is recommended for treatment of noninfectious epididymitis in patients on amiodarone therapy.

In children, Henoch-Schönlein Purpura, a small vessel vasculitis characterized by immunoglobulin A complex deposition, may also present with acute scrotum and vasculitic epididymitis. The disease typically occurs in children between 2 and 11 years old, presenting with palpable purpura, abdominal pain, hematuria, and joint pain. Scrotal swelling occurs in 2% to 38% of patients [38]. Ultrasound findings demonstrate findings consistent with epididymal inflammation, including epididymal enlargement, increased Doppler flow, scrotal skin thickening, and hydrocele. The disease is self-limiting and generally responsive to corticosteroid treatment. Once testicular torsion has been ruled out, awareness of the association of Henoch-Schönlein Purpura and scrotal pain should limit unnecessary surgical intervention in this population.

Chronic epididymitis

Chronic epididymitis, characterized by pain of at least 3 months in duration in the scrotum, testicle, or epididymis and localized to one or both epididymides on clinical examination, may account for up to 80% of patients presenting to the urology clinic with scrotal pain [3]. The average age at diagnosis of chronic epididymitis is 49 years, with the average patient having symptoms present for 5 years at the time of diagnosis [39]. Pain tends to be mild to moderate and typically does not affect daily activity, though chronic epididymal pain has a significant effect on quality of life, with 84% of patients describing quality of life as unsatisfying or terrible. Affected patients tend to have an increased number of sexual partners and a higher incidence of erectile dysfunction, musculoskeletal complaints, and neurologic disease compared with normal controls. Evaluation of patients with chronic epididymal pain should include assessment for chronic prostatitis and male pelvic pain syndrome, including prostatic fluid examination and careful evaluation for occult voiding dysfunction; however, patients with chronic epididymitis frequently have no history of documented infection or inciting event.

Diagnostic considerations

Although most diseases of the epididymis are benign, a thorough history and physical exam should always be performed to differentiate amongst epididymal pathology [17]. Patients presenting with a clinical diagnosis of epididymitis should undergo testing for the appropriate bacteria according to the Centers for Disease Control (CDC) guidelines (Box 1) [40]. Children and adolescents who are not sexually active should have urine obtained from a midstream urine collection, as should adults over the age of 35. Urine should be examined by urinary dipstick as well as microscopy. Patients with a positive dipstick or microscopy should have urine sent for definitive culture. In addition, patients with risk factors for complicated urinary tract infections such as those with recent urinary tract instrumentation, indwelling ureteral stents, or recent anal intercourse should also undergo urine culture for coliform bacteria. (Owing to increasing rates of antibiotic resistance, antibiotic sensitivities are routinely obtained at the authors' institution.)

Sexually active patients younger than 35 years old, as well as those over 35 with a new sexual

---

Box 1. Centers for Disease Control's 2006 guidelines for the diagnosis and management of epididymitis

Younger than 35
- Gram stain of urethral exudate for urethritis (>5 white blood cells/high power field) *or* leukocyte esterase test *or* microscopic examination of first-void urine sediment demonstrating at or above 10 WBC/hpf
- Culture or nucleic acid amplification test of urethral swab (or urine)
- Empiric antibiotics to cover *N gonnorheae* and *C trachomatis*
  — *Ceftriaxone 250 mg intramuscularly × 1
and
  — *Doxycycline 100 mg po bid × 10 days

Older than 35
- Leukocyte esterase test *or* microscopic examination of first-void urine sediment demonstrating at or above 10 WBC/hpf
- Culture and gram stain of voided urine
- Empiric antibiotics to cover coliform bacteria
  — Levofloxacin 500 mg qd × 10 days
or
  — Ofloxacin 300 mg bid × 10 days

---

* Patients younger than 35 with allergies to penicillins or tetracyclines should be treated with levofloxacin or ofloxacin.
* If *N gonnorheae* is suspected, patients may need to be desensitized to penicillin on account of the high rate of fluoroquinolone resistance evolving in *N gonnorheae*.

---

partner, should undergo testing for *C trachomatis*. In these instances, a gram-stained smear of urethral exudate or intraurethral swab specimen is indicated for diagnosis of urethritis (ie, ≥ 5 polymorphonuclear leukocytes per oil immersion field) and for presumptive diagnosis of gonococcal infection. If the urethral gram stain is negative, first-void uncentrifuged urine should be examined for leukocytes. Definitive diagnosis should be obtained on the basis of nucleic acid amplification tests such as polymerase chain reaction if available, as these tests have a greatly increased sensitivity for detection of *C trachomatis* over routine cultures [41]. Direct fluorescent antibody testing and optical immunoassay testing, although less sensitive than polymerase chain reaction, allow for rapid results that improve patient counseling and treatment. Patients with positive results for *C trachomatis* or *N gonorrhea* should be referred for further testing for other sexually transmitted diseases, including HIV, owing to an increased prevalence in this population.

Despite clear guidelines that have been in place for decades, epidemiologic studies of practice patterns reveal that both American and European physicians often do not follow established guidelines. In fact, for patients between the ages of 18 and 35, fewer than one third receive the appropriate diagnostic evaluation and fewer than half receive appropriate treatment according to established guidelines [42]. The explanation for why physicians do not follow guidelines is unknown, but may be the result of poor penetration of CDC guidelines into practice or a discordance between empiric experience and current guidelines.

Improvements in ultrasound technology, including higher megahertz transducers, has led to increased sensitivity and specificity in the evaluation of scrotal pathology. Although ultrasound is primarily used for ruling out torsion of the spermatic cord in cases of acute scrotum, it will often demonstrate epididymal hyperemia and swelling in patients with epididymitis. However, differentiation between testicular torsion and epididymitis is based on clinical evaluation, as partial spermatic cord torsion may mimic epididymitis on scrotal ultrasound [17]. Ultrasound of patients with a clear history consistent with epididymitis offers no diagnostic advantage: only 69% of patients with clinical epididymitis have a positive ultrasound, and a negative ultrasound does not alter physician management of clinical epididymitis [43]. Ultrasound, therefore, should be reserved for patients who have scrotal pain and no definitive diagnosis by physical exam, history, or objective laboratory findings.

Although rarely used because of advances in color-Doppler ultrasound, scrotal radionuclide scintigraphy may be used with a relatively high degree of sensitivity and specificity in differentiating testicular torsion from epididymitis in patients with acute scrotum [44]. A single bolus of $Na^{99}TcO_4-$ is injected intravenously and perfusion imaging is obtained at 2-second intervals for 2 minutes. A static image is performed after 10 minutes and compared with perfusion images.

In the nonpathologic scrotum, scrotal and testicular vessels are poorly visualized in the perfusion state, and the scrotum appears symmetric and homogeneous on static images. Patients with testicular torsion have an asymmetric decreased uptake in the affected testicle on perfusion imaging and decreased or absent uptake on static images. Conversely, patients with epididymitis have increased uptake of the radionuclide on perfusion and static images. Late torsion may elicit inflammatory changes that are confused with epididymitis.

Treatment

Treatment of epididymitis includes bed rest, scrotal elevation, analgesics, nonsteroidal anti-inflammatory drugs, and empiric antibiotics when infection is suspected. Although most patients can be treated on an outpatient basis, hospitalization may be considered if the patient appears toxic or has significant systemic findings (fever, leukocytosis, etc), or severe pain suggests other diagnoses (eg, torsion, testicular infarction, or necrotizing fasciitis). Additional consideration for admission should be given to patients with significant comorbidities, including severe immunosuppression or uncontrolled diabetes mellitus.

Antibiotics continue to be the primary treatment modality for epididymitis, despite evidence demonstrating that up to three quarters of patients do not have an identifiable bacterial infection [2,9]. Despite the fact that antibiotics do not alter the course of epididymitis in the absence of identifiable infection, the use of antibiotics has increased from 75% to 95% between 1965 and 2005 [2,9]. In 2007 the CDC published updated guidelines for the treatment of epididymitis, with the choice of antibiotics depending on patient age as well as history, including urinary tract instrumentation and sexual history (see Box 1). Patients who are younger than 35 or have a recent sexual risk factor are treated with a 10-day course of doxycycline as well as a single intramuscular injection of ceftriaxone to cover *N gonorrhea*. If patients are penicillin allergic, *C trachomatis* infections may be treated with levofloxacin or ofloxacin, but older quinolones such as ciprofloxacin should not be used on account of their incomplete coverage of *C trachomatis*. As of April 2007, the CDC no longer recommends use of fluoroquinolones to treat *N gonorrhea*, owing to an increasing prevalence of resistant organisms [40]. Therefore, patients with a suspected *N gonorrheal* infection should be treated with a single intramuscular dose of ceftriaxone in addition to doxycycline to cover *C trachomatis*. Patients with a cephalosporin allergy and fluoroquinolone-resistant *N gonorrhea* can be treated with spectinomycin (not available in United States) or undergo cephalosporin desensitization. Patients older than 35 and those with risk factors for enteric pathogens are treated with a quinolone antibiotic for 10 days [45]. Antibiotic sensitivities should be obtained in all patients with recent urinary tract instrumentation or risk factors for complicated urinary tract infections, as this population has higher rates of antibiotic resistance.

In patients where *C trachomatis* is confirmed or highly likely, consideration should be given to treating sexual partners. *C trachomatis* infections are a major cause of pelvic inflammatory disease, ectopic pregnancy, infertility, and chronic abdominal pain in women. In addition, continued infection of a partner may lead to recurrent infections and recurrent epididymitis. Partners may be treated directly, referred to their primary care physician for testing, or receive patient-delivered partner therapy, whereby the treating physician prescribes a second course of antibiotics that the patient then gives to his partner [46].

Atypical infections of the epididymis require specific treatment for the offending organism. Treatment of tuberculous epididymitis involves a 6-month triple drug course with isoniazid, rifampin, and pyrazinamide. Ethambutol should be added to the antimicrobial regimen while bacterial sensitivities are pending if the patient comes from an area with high drug resistance [47,48]. In contrast to patients with community-acquired TB, patients with Bacille Calmette-Guérin epididymitis should be treated with isoniazid and rifampin only, as all strains are resistant to pyrazinamide. Patients with *Brucella* epididymitis should be treated with 100-mg doxycycline orally twice daily for 6 weeks and either 1-gm streptomycin intramuscularly daily for 14 days or 600- to 900-mg rifampin orally daily for 6 weeks [49]. Treatment of filarial funiculoepididymitis consists of testis/cord-preserving surgical excision and use of diethylcarbamazine or ivermectin to control microfilaremia.

Although there are no specific studies regarding medical management of chronic epididymitis, reports of patients with orchalgia reveal that the use of local therapy (heat), nerve blocks, analgesics, anti-inflammatories, or drugs such as tricyclics and anticonvulsants (gabapentin) are rarely effective, largely empirical, and not supported by randomized placebo controlled trials [50]. Medical management, therefore, must rely on a combination of therapies with effectiveness often being patient specific.

Attempts at treatment of idiopathic epididymal pain should begin with use of a long-acting anti-inflammatory agent, such as naproxen sodium, given on a daily basis for at least 2 weeks. Anti-inflammatories should be given in conjunction with limiting patient activity as well as scrotal ice and elevation. If the patient fails to have relief from these measures, the use of a tricyclic antidepressant or a neuroleptic such as gabapentin should be considered, with selection based on any other comorbidities. Patients who do not respond to a several-month course of one of these centrally acting medications may be considered for spermatic cord block using a mixture of 6-mL 1% plain lidocaine along with 1 mL of methylprednisolone (40 mg/mL). Despite these multiple therapies, the vast majority of patients may continue to have substantial discomfort and may be considered for chronic pain management with narcotics and referral to a chronic pain specialist [39].

Epididymectomy has high failure rates (>75%) in the treatment of chronic epididymitis owing to plasticity in circuits involved in central pain processing [51]. Transient relief following surgery is often followed by either recurrence of pain or transfer of symptoms to the contralateral epididymis. In addition, epididymectomy may be associated with infertility or testicular loss intra-operatively or from subsequent atrophy. Orchiectomy may be considered in patients with unrelenting epididymal pain that significantly affects their quality of life, though up to 50% of patients may continue to have scrotal pain [50]. Patients should undergo extensive conservative management as well as psychologic evaluation before consideration of orchiectomy for chronic orchalgia, and the surgeon should be aware of the medical legal aspects of this radical procedure, which may fail to achieve its goal in a significant number of patients.

Summary

Epididymitis affects a large cross section of the population. There are several causes of epididymal inflammation: infection, trauma, autoimmune disease, vasculitis, and idiopathic. Epididymitis should be further classified as acute (< 6 weeks) or chronic, with evaluation and treatment based on duration of symptoms. Diagnosis is determined based on clinical history and studies for evaluation of urinary tract infection, with imaging modalities reserved for distinguishing torsion of the spermatic cord. Although classically thought of as an infectious process, the majority of men in large epidemiologic studies have no demonstrable infection. CDC guidelines outline the current approach to the evaluation and treatment of acute infectious epididymitis, though guidelines are often not followed. Treatment of chronic epididymitis is difficult, and treatment must be based on individual response to therapy following a stepwise treatment plan. Additional research into the etiology and treatment of this common urologic condition is warranted and may alter future treatment guidelines.

References

[1] Collins MM, Stafford RS, O'Leary MP, et al. How common is prostatitis? A national survey of physician visits. J Urol 1998;159:1224–8.

[2] Tracy CR, Costabile RA. The changing face of epididymitis from 1965 to 2005. Abstract presentation, 53rd James C. Kimbrough Urological Seminar, Savannah, GA. January 16, 2006.

[3] Nickel JC, Teichman JM, Gregoire M, et al. Prevalence, diagnosis, characterization, and treatment of prostatitis, interstitial cystitis, and epididymitis in outpatient urologic practice: the Canadian PIE Study. Urology 2005;66:935–40.

[4] Moore CA, Lockett BL, Lennox KW, et al. Prednisone in the treatment of acute epididymitis: a cooperative study. J Urol 1971;106: 578–80.

[5] Hoppner W, Strohmeyer T, Hartmann Lopez-Gamarra D, et al. Surgical treatment of acute epididymitis and its underlying diseases. Eur Urol 1992;22: 218–21.

[6] Ludwig M, Johannes S, Bergmann M, et al. Experimental Escherichia coli epididymitis in rats: a model to assess the outcome of antibiotic treatment. Br J Urol 2002;73:933–8.

[7] See W, Taylor T, Mack L, et al. Bacteria; epididymitis in the rat: a model for assessing the impact of acute inflammation on epididymal antibiotic penetration. J Urol 1990;144:780–3.

[8] Jantos C, Baumgartner W, Durchfield B, et al. Experimental epididymitis due to Chlamydia trachomatis in rats. Infect Immun 1992;60(6):2324–8.

[9] Mittemeyer BT, Lennox KW, Borski AA. Epididymitis: a review of 610 cases. J Urol 1966;95:390–2.

[10] Berger RE, Alexander ER, Harnisch JP, et al. Etiology, manifestations, and therapy of acute epididymitis: prospective study of 50 cases. J Urol 1979;121: 750–4.

[11] Schmidt SS, Hinman F. The effect of vasectomy upon the incidence of epididymitis after prostatectomy: an analysis of 810 operations. J Urol 1950; 63(2):872–81.

[12] Hawkins DA, Taylor-Robinson D, Thomas BJ, et al. Microbiological survey of acute epididymitis. Genitourin Med 1986;62:342–4.

[13] Scheibel JH, Anderson JT, Brandenhoff P, et al. Chlamydia trachomatis in acute epididymitis. Scand J Urol Nephrol 1983;17:47–50.

[14] Pearson RC, Baumber CD, McGhie D, et al. The relevance of Chlamydia trachomatis in acute epididymitis in young men. Br J Urol 1988;62:72–5.

[15] Grant JF, Costello CB, Sequeira PJ, et al. The role of Chlamydia trachomatis in epididymitis. Br J Urol 1987;60:355–9.

[16] Melekos M, Asbach H. Epididymitis: aspects concerning etiology and treatment. J Urol 1987;138: 83–6.

[17] Tracy CR, Steers WD. Anatomy, physiology and diseases of the epididymis. AUA Update Series 2007; XXVI: lesson 12.

[18] Somekh E, Gorenstein A, Serour F. Acute epididymitis in boys: evidence of a post-infectious etiology. J Urol 2004;171(1):391–4.

[19] Lau P, Anderson PA, Giacomantonio JM, et al. Acute epididymitis in boys: are antibiotics indicated? Br J Urol 1997;79:797–800.

[20] Ulbright TM, Amin MB, Young RH. Miscellaneous primary tumors of the testis, adnexa, and spermatic cord. In: Rosai J, Sobin LH, editors. Atlas of tumor pathology, fasc 25, ser 3. Washington, DC: Armed Forces Institute of Pathology; 1999. p. 235–66.

[21] Heaton ND, Hogan B, Mitchell M, et al. Tuberculous epididymo-orchitis: clinical and ultrasound observations. Br J Urol 1989;64:305–9.

[22] Menke JJ, Heins JR. Epididymo-orchits following intravesical bacillus calmette-guerin therapy. Ann Pharmacother 2000;34:479–82.

[23] Ferrie BG, Rundle JS. Tuberculous epidiymo-orchitis. A review of 20 cases. Br J Urol 1983;55:437–9.

[24] Pappas G, Akritidis N, Bostilkovski M, et al. Brucellosis. N Engl J Med 2005;352:2325–36.

[25] Troy SB, Rickman LS, Davis CE. Brucellosis in San Diego: epidemiology and species-related differences in acute clinical presentations. Medicine (Baltimore) 2005;84:174–87.

[26] Ozturk A, Ozturk E, Zeyrek F, et al. Comparison of brucella and non-specific epididymorchitis: grey scale and color Doppler ultrasonographic features. Eur J Radiol 2005;56:256–62.

[27] Williams PB, Henderson RJ, Sanusi ID, et al. Ultrasound diagnosis of filarial funiculoepididymitis. Urology 1996;48(4):644–6.

[28] Christiansen CG, Sandlow JI. Testicular pain following vasectomy: a review of post-vasectomy pain syndrome. J Androl 2003;24(3):293–8.

[29] Ryan DM, Lesser BA, Crumley LA, et al. Epididymal sarcoidosis. J Urol 1993;149(1):134–6.

[30] Burke BJ, Parker SH, Hopper KD, et al. The ultra-sonographic appearance of coexistent epididymal and testicular sarcoidosis. J Clin Ultrasound 1990; 18:522–6.

[31] Forte MD, Brant WE. Ultrasonographic detection of epididymal sarcoidosis. J Clin Ultrasound 1988; 16:191–4.

[32] Suzuki Y, Koike H, Tamura G, et al. Ultrasono-graphic findings of epididymal sarcoidosis. Urol Int 1994;52:228–30.

[33] Rudin L, Megalli M, Mesa-Tejada R. Genital sar-coidosis. Urology 1974;3(6):750–4.

[34] Svetec DA, Waguespack RL, Sabanegh ES Jr. In-termittent azoospermia associated with epididymal sarcoidosis. Fertil Steril 1998;70(4):777–9.

[35] Cho YH, Lee KH, Band D, et al. Clinical features of patients with Behcet's disease and epididymitis. J Urol 2003;170(4):1231–3.

[36] Greene HL, Graham EL, Werner JA, et al. Toxic and therapeutic effects of amiodarone in the treat-ment of cardiac arrhythmias. J Am Coll Cardiol 1983;2(6):1114–28.

[37] Gasparich JP, Mason JT, Greene HL, et al. Amio-darone-associated epididymitis: drug-related epidid-ymitis in the absence of infection. J Urol 1985; 133(6):971–2.

[38] Huang LH, Yeung CY, Shyur SD, et al. Diagnosis of Henoch-Schonlein purpura by soography and nu-clear scanning in a child presenting with bilateral acute scrotum. J Microbiol Immunol Infect 2004; 37:192–5.

[39] Nickel CJ, Siemens RD, Nickel KR, et al. The patient with chronic epididymitis: characterization of an enigmatic syndrome. J Urol 2002;167:1701.

[40] Workowski KA, Berman SM. Sexually transmitted diseases treatment guidelines, 2006. MMWR Rec-ommendations and reports. Aug 2006. 55(RR11): 1-94. Available at: www.cdc.gov/std/treatment.

[41] Swain GR, McDonald RA, Pfister JR, et al. Decision analysis: point of care chlamydia testing vs. labora-tory-based methods. Clin Med Res 2004;2(1):29–35.

[42] Drury NE, Dyer JP, Breitenfeldt N, et al. Manage-ment of acute epididymitis: are European guidelines being followed? Eur Urol 2004;46:522–5.

[43] Tracy CR, Witmer MT, Costabile RA. The use of ul-trasound in patients with clinical epididymitis in a university-based health care system. Poster presen-tation, 65th Annual Mid-Atlantic Section of AUA. Southampton, Bermuda, October 18–21, 2008.

[44] Yuon Z, Luo Q, Chen L, et al. Clinical study of scro-tum scintigraphy in 49 patients with acute scrotal pain: a comparison with ultrasonography. Ann Nucl Med 2001;15(3):225–30.

[45] Eickhoff JH, Frimodt-Moller N, Frimodt-Moller C. A double blind randomized controlled multicentre study to compare the efficacy of Ciprofloxacin with Pavampicillin as oral therapy for epididymitis in men over 40 years of age. BJU Int 1999;84(7): 827–34.

[46] Packel LJ, Guerry S, Bauer HM, et al. Patient-deliv-ered partner therapy for chlamydial infections: atti-tudes and practices of California physicians and nurse practitioners. Sex Transm Dis 2006;33(7): 458–63.

[47] Hinzes JD, Winn RE. Tuberculosis of the urogenital tract. Infectious diseases. 2nd edition. Mosby: An Imprint of Elsevier; 2004. p. 773–7.

[48] Al-Ghazo MA, Bani-Hani KE, Amarin ZO. Tuber-culous epididymitis and fertility in North Jordan. Saudi Med J 2005;26(8):1212–5.

[49] Solera J, Geijo P, Largo J, et al. Grupo de Estu-dio de Castilla-la Mancha de Enfermedades Infec-ciosas. A randomized, double-blind study to assess the optimal duration of doxycycline treat-ment for human brucellosis. Clin Infect Dis 2004;39(12):1776–82.

[50] Davis BE, Noble MJ. Analysis and management of chronic orchalgia. AUA Update Series 1992; XI: lesson 2.

[51] Padmore DE, Norman RW, Millard OH. Analyses of indications for and outcomes of epididymectomy. J Urol 1996;156(1):95–6.

ELSEVIER
SAUNDERS

Urol Clin N Am 35 (2007) 109–115

UROLOGIC CLINICS
of North America

Inflammation and Benign Prostatic Hyperplasia

J. Curtis Nickel, MD

Department of Urology, Queen's University, Kingston, Ontario, Canada

Prostatitis, a histologic diagnosis, has evolved over the years to describe a clinical syndrome that was believed to be associated with prostatic inflammation. Similarly, benign prostatic hyperplasia (BPH), another histologic diagnosis, has evolved to describe a clinical syndrome believed to be associated with prostatic enlargement. Recent explorations of the interrelationships between these prostate-associated histologic and clinical conditions have generated much interest and excitement. This article describes these relationships and their impact on the management of, in particular, BPH.

Definitions

BPH is correctly defined as enlargement of the prostate gland from the progressive hyperplasia of stromal and glandular prostatic cells [1]. Clinical BPH refers to the lower urinary tract symptoms (LUTS) associated with benign prostatic enlargement (BPE) causing bladder outlet obstruction (BOO). Clinical prostatitis can be divided into acute and chronic bacterial prostatitis (National Institutes of Health [NIH] Categories I and II), rare infectious diseases of the prostate gland, the much more common chronic prostatitis/chronic pelvic pain syndrome (Category III CP/CPPS), and asymptomatic inflammatory prostatitis (Category IV) [2]. Histologic prostatitis refers to the confirmation of prostate inflammation by microscopic examination. Asymptomatic prostate

Dr. Nickel's prostatitis and benign prostatic hyperplasia (BPH) research are funded in part by grants from the National Institutes of Health/National Institute of Diabetes and Digestive and Kidney Diseases: NIH/NIDDK DK065174 (prostatitis), NIH/NIDDK DK063797 (BPH).

E-mail address: jcn@queensu.ca

inflammation would be categorized as Category IV. Table 1 presents definitions and classifications of these various BPH and prostatitis conditions.

Lack of association of histologic prostatitis and clinical prostatitis

Traditionally, prostatitis has referred to a clinical condition associated with infection and/or inflammation of the prostate. The clinical diagnosis of a symptomatic prostatitis syndrome is made on the basis of clinical symptoms, some clinical findings, culture results, and in some cases, demonstration of inflammation in prostate fluid (expressed prostatic secretions or postprostatic massage urine). Although this concept does hold true for bacterial prostatitis (Categories I and II) confirmed with specific bacterial cultures, it may not be as simple in the much more common Category III CP/CPPS.

An examination of the 488 men enrolled in the NIH-Chronic Prostatitis Cohort (CPC) study determined that leukocytes in the prostate-specific specimens (expressed prostatic secretions [EPS] or postprostatic massage urine specimens [VB3]) did not correlate with any specific symptoms or symptom severity [3]. The inflammatory status (leukocyte counts in EPS and/or VB3) in a total of 463 men enrolled in the NIH CPC study were compared with 121 age-matched control men without any urinary or pain symptoms [4]. Men with CP/CPPS had significantly higher leukocyte counts in these specimens (50% and 32% had 5 or more, or 10 or more white blood cells per high power field in EPS, respectively) than asymptomatic men (40% and 20%, respectively). The high prevalence of leukocytes in the asymptomatic control population certainly raised questions about the clinical relevance of inflammation detected by current diagnostic tools. A small-scale

Table 1
Definitions and categorization of histologic and clinical benign prostatic hyperplasia and prostatitis

Type	Benign prostatic hyperplasia		Prostatitis	
	Histologic	Clinical	Histologic	Clinical
Definition	Enlargement of the prostate gland from the progressive hyperplasia of prostatic cells	The lower urinary tract symptoms associated with BPE	Microscopic evidence of prostate inflammation	Prostate/pelvic pain syndrome
Subcategories	Glandular stromal	LUTS BPE BOO	Acute Chronic	Cat I–acute bacterial Cat II–chronic bacterial Cat III–chronic pelvic pain syndrome

Abbreviations: BOO, bladder outlet obstruction; BPE, benign prostatic enlargement; LUTS, lower urinary tract symptoms.

study [5], which examined correlations between the symptoms and histology of prostatitis in biopsies of men with a clinical diagnosis of CP/CPPS, suggested that histologic inflammation may not be a significant factor in the disease process. Of the 97 patients examined, just 33% had histologic evidence of inflammation, with only 5% having a moderate or severe grading.

An examination of 5597 men with biopsy and clinical evaluation of prostatitis-like symptoms (completion of chronic prostatitis symptom index [CPSI]) enrolled in the REduction by DUtasteride of prostate Cancer Events (REDUCE) study [6] provides the largest body of data examining relationships between symptoms of CP and histologic prostate inflammation. The study population consisted of aging men with elevated levels of prostate-specific antigen (PSA), but with a negative prostate cancer biopsy, recruited as an "at-risk" group for the development of prostate cancer [6]. Chronic histologic inflammation was found in more than 78% of men in REDUCE [7], reflecting its almost ubiquitous nature in aging men. Acute inflammation was found in 16.5% of the study population, and when present was almost always graded as mild. Data from this analysis of REDUCE population failed to establish substantive links between the CPSI and the presence of histologic inflammation. In men with acute inflammation, no correlations between total or component CPSI scores, including presence of prostatitis-like symptom complex, and inflammation were observed. For those with chronic inflammation, a weak but statistically significant association was observed between inflammation status and total CPSI score, but no significant relationships with pain were observed. From

a clinical perspective, presence of chronic prostatitis-like symptoms did not provide any discriminative value for a histologic diagnosis of either acute or chronic inflammation.

Association of clinical prostatitis and benign prostatic hyperplasia

BPH is a disease of aging men: an estimated 42% of men 51 to 60 years of age have histologic BPH [1]. The incidence increases to more than 70% in men 61 to 70 years of age and to almost 90% in those 81 to 90 years of age. The prevalence of LUTS associated with BPH parallels that of pathologic BPH; more than 50% of men over 50 are believed to experience LUTS secondary to an enlarged prostate gland.

Prostatitis has traditionally been considered a condition that afflicts younger men, but it is apparent that it is as common in older men [8]. Compared with men 51 years and older, the odds of a documented prostatitis diagnosis is only twofold greater in younger men [9]. Approximately 8% of men over 50 report at least some mild prostatitis-like symptom in the past week compared with 11% of younger men [10]. Little attention has been given to the association between BPH and prostatitis, despite the high prevalence of both conditions in aging men.

Many physicians have trouble clinically distinguishing prostatitis from BPH in the older male population [11]. In 1992, 31,681 United States health professionals without prostate cancer provided information on urologic diagnoses and lower urinary tract symptoms [12]. Of the 5053 men with prostatitis, 57.2% also reported a history of BPH, whereas 38.7% of the 7465 men with BPH reported a history of prostatitis.

Clinical BPH is characterized by voiding LUTS. Prostatitis is characterized primarily by pain. Pain and/or discomfort on ejaculation is one of the most common and bothersome symptoms, but also the most differentiating symptom experienced by men with CP [13]. Painful ejaculation has been reported by approximately 5% to 31% of men with LUTS related to BPH in both community and clinic populations [14–18].

There is no doubt that the clinical syndromes of prostatitis and BPH can coexist, but is the diagnosis of clinical prostatitis at a young age a risk factor for development of later BPH? A population-based sample of 2447 men residing in Olmsted County, Minnesota, was evaluated to determine whether physician-diagnosed or self-reported prostatitis was associated with development of clinical BPH or related outcomes [19]. Physician-diagnosed prostatitis was associated with a 2.4-fold increase in the odds of receiving a later diagnosis of BPH. Men with a history of prostatitis were also more likely to receive treatment for BPH compared with men without prostatitis. A diagnosis of prostatitis may be an early marker for later development of BPH.

Association of inflammation and clinical benign prostatic hyperplasia

Histologic inflammation can be demonstrated in the majority of BPH pathologic specimens [20–23]. For years, the importance and clinical relevance of these seemingly asymptomatic inflammatory infiltrates were only speculated on.

REDUCE is an ongoing, large-scale, 4-year clinical study designed to determine whether and to what extent the dual 5α reductase inhibitor dutasteride reduces the risk of biopsy-detectable prostate cancer compared with placebo in men at high risk of developing prostate cancer [6]. The entrance criteria for the REDUCE study included the requirement of a prostate cancer-negative biopsy before enrollment. The data from the entrance biopsy have enabled additional protocol-defined investigations to be made, including examination of the baseline relationships between histologic prostate inflammation and LUTS, as measured with the International Prostate Symptom Score (IPSS) in over 8000 men. Using a modification of the histologic classification of prostatitis proposed by Nickel and colleagues

[24], a central pathology laboratory (Bostwick Laboratories, Richmond, VA) graded average acute and chronic inflammation across all biopsy cores on a 4-point scale (none, 0; mild, 1; moderate, 2; marked, 3) based on average cell density and extent of tissue involvement in each biopsy core.

Given that the mean prostate volume in men enrolled in the REDUCE study [6] was 46 mL and the PSA 5.8 ng/mL, it is likely that histologic BPH is common in the REDUCE population. As would be expected, chronic histologic inflammation was found in more than 78% of men in REDUCE [25]. Statistically significant but clinically small increases in IPSS symptoms were noted in men with inflammation compared with those without (eg, Wilcoxon rank-sum test for differences in total IPSS by presence versus absence of maximum chronic inflammation unadjusted, $P < .0001$). Similarly, statistically significant correlations were found between average chronic inflammation score and the IPSS variables. However, the magnitude of these correlations was small, indicating very weak associations. The clinical relevance of the small, but statistically significant difference in IPSS in patients with and without chronic inflammation and the statistically significant, but weak associations between chronic inflammation and IPSS demonstrates a consistent pattern—namely, that inflammation in BPH may be important.

If inflammation is indeed associated with BPH symptoms, anti-inflammatory agents should be investigated as new targets for the pharmacologic treatment of BPH. Given that nonsteroidal anti-inflammatory drugs are well known for their ability to decrease pain and inflammation, the effectiveness of ibuprofen together with the alpha-blocker, doxazosin, on BPH was evaluated for their efficacy in decreasing the expression of JM-27, a protein particularly expressed in the prostate that appears to be highly up-regulated in symptomatic BPH [26]. This study showed that doxazosin, as well as ibuprofen, significantly decreased cell viability and induced apoptosis in BPH prostate cell lines. In addition, it decreased the expression of JM-27. Unfortunately, there are few good data available to assess the clinical response of anti-inflammatory therapy in BPH. A single-center, unblinded trial randomized 46 men with LUTS and BPH to receive rofecoxib (a COX-2 inhibitor) 25 mg/day plus finasteride 5 mg/day versus finasteride 5 mg/day alone for 24 weeks [27]. The study found that, although there was not a significant difference between symptom improvement at 24 weeks, there was a statistically significant advantage of the combination therapy compared with finasteride alone in a short-term interval (4 weeks). It was hypothesized that the association of rofecoxib with finasteride induced a more rapid improvement in clinical results until the effect of finasteride becomes predominant. Phytotherapy has become one of the most popular treatment modalities for BPH. One of the primary mechanisms of why these herbal agents work is the anti-inflammatory effects of the various herbal preparations [28].

Role of inflammation in the pathogenesis of histologic benign prostatic hyperplasia

Three recent reviews on the pathogenesis of BPH have provided an evidence-based thesis that strongly suggests a role of inflammation in the propagation of histologic BPH [29–31]. Kramer and Marberger [31] recently outlined the current state of knowledge in regard to the influence of inflammation on the pathogenesis of BPH. Chronic inflammatory infiltrates, mainly composed of chronically activated T cells and macrophages, frequently are associated with BPH nodules [20,32,33]. These infiltrating cells are responsible for the production of cytokines (IL-2 and IFNγ), which may support fibromuscular growth in BPH [34]. Immigration of T cells into the area is attracted by increased production of pro-inflammatory cytokines such as IL-6, IL-8, and IL-15 [29,30,35]. Surrounding cells become targets and are killed (unknown mechanisms), leaving behind vacant spaces that are replaced by fibromuscular nodules with a specific pattern of a Th0/Th3 type of immune response [36].

What is not known is why the leukocyte population increases in BPH. A number of hypotheses have been generated based on recent basic research. In-situ studies demonstrated elevated expression of pro-inflammatory cytokines in BPH. IL-6, IL-8, and IL-17 may perpetuate chronic immune response in BPH and induce fibromuscular growth by an autocrine or paracrine loop [36,37] or via induction of COX-2 expression [38]. Immune reaction may be activated via Toll-like receptor signaling and mediated by macrophages and T cells [37]. Conversely, anti-inflammatory factors such as macrophage inhibitory cytokine-1 [39] may be decreased in symptomatic BPH tissues. Animal models provided

evidence for the presence of unique T-cell subsets that may suppress autoimmunity in healthy Sprague–Dawley rats resistant to chronic nonbacterial prostatitis [40]. On the basis of the available scientific evidence, it is highly likely that age-dependent weakening of the immune system, coupled with modified hormonal secretion, leads to the deterioration of a postulated population of suppressor cells that actively suppresses the recognition of prostatic antigens, leading to gradual infiltration of the prostate by lymphocytes and subsequent cascade of events that leads to BPH [41].

Impact of inflammation on progression of clinical benign prostatic hyperplasia

An examination of baseline prostate biopsies in a subgroup of 1197 patients in the Medical Therapies of Prostatic Symptoms study found that there was a chronic inflammatory infiltrate in 43% of the men [42]. It was hypothesized that the presence of histologic inflammation may be a predictor of progression. There was a highly clinically significant difference in the progression rate based on the presence or absence of inflammation. Patients in all groups (placebo, finasteride, doxazosin, and combination finasteride and doxazosin) with inflammation were more likely to progress clinically in terms of symptoms, acute urinary retention (AUR), or BPH-related surgery. For those with no inflammation, there was overall clinical progression in 13.2% of patients, whereas 3.9% had BPH-related surgery and none had AUR; corresponding values for those who had chronic inflammation were 21% ($P = .08$ versus no inflammation), 7.3% (not significant), and 5.6% ($P = .003$). Chronic inflammation accounted for every AUR event in this subgroup of patients with prostate biopsies, whereas in patients with no inflammation, there was no AUR.

The observation that the presence of prostatic inflammation may be clinically relevant in terms of prediction of BPH-related progression is very important. The 4-year longitudinal follow-up of the 8000 men enrolled in the REDUCE study [6,7,25] may confirm this finding. Many of these men would have had BPH at baseline (predicted by baseline high mean IPSS scores, elevated PSA, and negative initial biopsy). The baseline histologic status of these men are documented, and progression data in terms of BPH symptom and event (surgery and AUR) progression will be collected. A further important point is that inflammation may also have an important role in the pathogenesis of prostate cancer (see the article by Siemens elsewhere in this issue for further exploration of this topic), and that particular association will become clear when the REDUCE study is completed.

Biomarkers for inflammation in benign prostatic hyperplasia

If inflammation is associated with the pathogenesis, symptoms, and progression of BPH, a biomarker would be invaluable. There are a number of early candidates, and many others are currently being assessed by international research groups.

A small study [43] suggested that measurement of serum malondialdehyde, an index of inflammation and oxidative stress, may be a useful marker in BPH. Serum malondialdehyde levels analyzed in 22 BPH patients and 22 healthy donors showed an increase in levels in the BPH patients and a positive correlation with PSA (used here as a marker of prostate hyperplasia). It is not known whether this association has been replicated.

The association of serum C-reactive protein concentration—a nonspecific marker of inflammation—and LUTS, suggestive of BPH, was examined in 2337 men who participated in the Third National Health and Nutrition Examination Survey between 1988 and 1994 [44]. The survey found that men with a C-reactive protein concentration above the limit of detection (>3.00 mg/L) were 1.47 times more likely to have three or more symptoms than men with a C-reactive protein concentration below the detection limit (not statistically significant).

Cytokines, chemokines, and inflammatory mediators are believed to be important in the pathogenesis of prostate inflammation. Increased expression of IL-8 is noted in BPH tissue culture [45], which by direct and indirect mechanisms could promote proliferation of nonsenescent epithelial and stromal cells, thus contributing to the increased tissue growth seen in BPH. Such processes may lead to the discovery of potential biomarkers for prostate inflammation in BPH. Seminal plasma levels of eight cytokines and nine chemokines were evaluated in 83 men: 20 healthy controls, 9 with CP/CPPS IIIA (inflammatory), 31 with CP/CPPS IIIB (non-inflammatory), and 23 with BPH [46]. Prostate specimens from 13 BPH patients were analyzed to detect IL-8–producing cells and to characterize inflammatory infiltrates. IL-8 concentration in seminal plasma was positively correlated with symptom scores in both the CP/CPPS patients and BPH patients.

Although a number of potential markers (C-reactive protein, IL-8, markers of oxidative stress) have been evaluated, these markers are generally

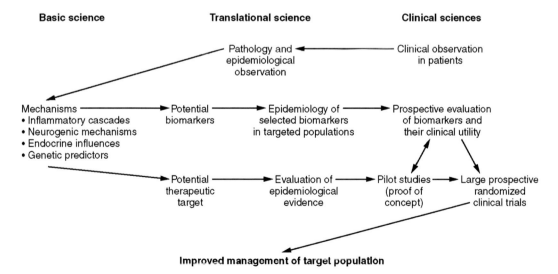

Fig. 1. A bidirectional translational research approach (bench to bedside) will eventually improve the understanding of the association of inflammation with BPH and result in better stratification of patients for risk assessment and focused treatment.

nonspecific for prostate or BPH. However, it opens the search for biomarkers that could be used to stratify patients as to risk of developing BPH or related BPH adverse outcomes, or to monitor symptoms and response to medical therapy for BPH.

Summary

Inflammation in the prostate gland appears to be more closely related to BPH than the clinical syndrome CP. A translational approach to research (bed to bedside) should unlock the mysteries of this association (Fig. 1). Further understanding of the role of inflammation in BPH and clinical detection of this inflammation will expand the understanding of BPH pathogenesis and its histologic and clinical progression, allow risk stratification for patients presenting with BPH-related LUTS, and suggest novel treatment strategies.

References

[1] Berry SJ, Coffey DS, Walsh PC, et al. The development of human benign prostatic hyperplasia with age. J Urol 1984;132:474–9.

[2] Krieger JN, Nyberg L, Nickel JC. NIH consensus definition and classification of prostatitis. JAMA 1999;282:236–7.

[3] Schaeffer AJ, Knauss JS, Landis JR, et al. Leukocyte and bacterial counts do not correlate with severity of symptoms in men with chronic prostatitis: the NIH chronic prostatitis cohort (CPC) study. J Urol 2002;168(3):1048–53.

[4] Nickel JC, Alexander RB, Schaeffer AJ, et al. Leukocytes and bacteria in men with chronic prostatitis/chronic pelvic pain syndrome compared to asymptomatic controls. J Urol 2003;170(3):818–22.

[5] True LD, Berger RE, Rothman I, et al. Prostate histopathology and the chronic prostatitis/chronic pelvic pain syndrome: a prospective biopsy study. J Urol 1999;162:2014–8.

[6] Andriole G, Bostwick D, Brawley O, et al. Chemoprevention of prostate cancer in men at high risk: rationale and design of the reduction by dutasteride of prostate cancer events (REDUCE) trial. J Urol 2004;172:1314–7.

[7] Nickel JC, Roehrborn CG, O'Leary MP, et al. Examination of the relationship between symptoms of prostatitis and histologic inflammation: baseline data from the REDUCE chemoprevention trial. J Urol 2007;178:896–901.

[8] Pontari MA. Chronic prostatitis/chronic pelvic pain syndrome in elderly men: toward better understanding and treatment. Drugs Aging 2003;20:1111–25.

[9] Roberts RO, Lieber MM, Rhodes T, et al. Prevalence of a physician-assigned diagnosis of prostatitis: the Olmsted County Study of Urinary Symptoms and Health Status Among Men. Urology 1998;51: 578–84.

[10] Nickel JC, Downey J, Hunter D, et al. Prevalence of prostatitis-like symptoms in a population based study using the National Institutes of Health Chronic Prostatitis Symptom Index. J Urol 2001; 165:842–5.

[11] Collins MM, Stafford RS, O'Leary MP, et al. Distinguishing chronic prostatitis and benign prostatic hyperplasia symptoms: results of a national survey of physician visits. Urology 1999;53:921–5.

[12] Collins MM, Meigs JB, Barry MJ, et al. Prevalence and correlates of prostatitis in the health professionals follow-up study cohort. J Urol 2002;167(3): 1363–6.

[13] Shoskes DA, Landis JR, Wang Y, et al. Impact of post-ejaculatory pain in men with category III chronic prostatitis/chronic pelvic pain syndrome. J Urol 2004;172:542–7.

[14] Vallancien G, Emberton M, Harving N, et al. Sexual dysfunction in 1,274 European men suffering from lower urinary tract symptoms. J Urol 2003;169(6): 2257–61.

[15] Frankel SJ, Donovan JL, Peters TJ, et al. Sexual dysfunction in men with lower urinary tract symptoms. J Clin Epidemiol 1998;51(8):677–85.

[16] Brookes SJ, Donovan JL, Peters TJ, et al. Sexual dysfunction in men after treatment for lower urinary tract symptoms: evidence from randomized control trial. Br Med J 2002;324:1059–61.

[17] Rosen R, Altwein J, Boyle P, et al. Lower urinary tract symptoms and male sexual dysfunction: the multinational survey of the aging male (MSAM-7). Eur Urol 2003;44:637–49.

[18] Nickel JC, Elhilali M, Vallancien G for the ALF-ONE Study Group. Benign prostatic hyperplasia (BPH) and prostatitis: prevalence of painful ejaculation in men with clinical BPH. BJU Int 2005;95: 571–4.

[19] St. Sauver JL, Jacobson DJ, McGree ME, et al. Association between prostatitis and development of benign prostatic hyperplasia. J Urol 2007; 177(Suppl 4):497 (abstract 1506).

[20] Kohnen PW, Drach GW. Patterns of inflammation in prostatic hyperplasia: a histologic and bacteriologic study. J Urol 1979;121:755–60.

[21] Nickel JC. Prostatic inflammation in benign prostatic hyperplasia—the third component? Can J Urol 1994;1(1):1–4.

[22] Odunjo EO, Elebute EA. Chronic prostatitis in benign prostatic hyperplasia. Br J Urol 1971;43:333–7.

[23] Nickel JC, Downey J, Young I, et al. Asymptomatic inflammation and/or infection in benign prostatic hyperplasia. BJU Int 1999;84:976–81.

[24] Nickel JC, True LD, Kreiger JN, et al. Consensus development of a histopathological classification system for chronic prostatic inflammation. BJU Int 2001;87:797–805.

[25] Nickel JC, Roehrborn CG, O'Leary MP, et al. The relationship between prostate inflammation and lower urinary tract symptoms: examination of baseline data from the REDUCE trial. J Urol 2007; 177(Suppl 4):34–5 (abstract 98).

[26] Minnery CH, Getzenberg RH. Benign prostatic hyperplasia cell line viability and modulation of JM-27 by Doxazosin and Ibuprofen. J Urol 2005;174:375–9.

[27] Di Silverio F, Bosman C, Slavatori M, et al. Combination therapy with rofecoxib and finasteride in the treatment of men with lower urinary tract symptoms (LUTS) and benign prostatic hyperplasia (BPH). Eur Urol 2005;47:72–9.

[28] Buck AC. Is there a scientific basis for the therapeutic effects of serenoa repens in benign prostatic hyperplasia? Mechanisms of action. J Urol 2004;172:1792–9.

[29] Lee KL, Peehl DM. Molecular and cellular pathogenesis of benign prostatic hyperplasia. J Urol 2004;172:1784–91.

[30] Untergasser G, Madersbacher S, Berger P. Benign prostatic hyperplasia: age-related tissue-remodeling. Exp Gerontol 2005;40:121–8.

[31] Kramer G, Marberger M. Could inflammation be a key component in the progression of benign prostatic hyperplasia? Curr Opin Urol 2006;16:25–9.

[32] Theyer G, Kramer G, Assmann I. Phenotypic characterization of infiltrating leukocytes in benign prostatic hyperplasia. Lab Invest 1992;66:96–107.

[33] Steiner G, Gessl A, Kramer G, et al. Phenotype and function of peripheral and prostatic lymphocytes in patients with benign prostatic hyperplasia. J Urol 1994;151:480–4.

[34] Kramer G, Steiner GE, Handisurya A, et al. Increased expression of lymphocyte-derived cytokines in benign hyperplastic prostate tissue, identification of the producing cell types, and effect of differentially expressed cytokines on stromal cell proliferation. Prostate 2002;52:43–8.

[35] Handisurya A, Steiner GE, Stix U, et al. Differential expression of interleukin-15, a pro-inflammatory cytokine and T-cell growth factor, and its receptor in human prostate. Prostate 2001;49:251–62.

[36] Steiner G, Stix U, Handisurya A, et al. Cytokine expression pattern in benign prostatic hyperplasia infiltrating T cells and impact of lymphocytic infiltration on cytokine mRNA profile in prostatic tissue. Lab Invest 2003;83:1131–46.

[37] Konig JE, Senge T, Allhoff EP, et al. Analysis of the inflammatory network in benign prostate hyperplasia and prostate cancer. Prostate 2004;58:121–9.

[38] Wang W, Bergh A, Damber JE. Chronic inflammation in benign prostate hyperplasia is associated with focal upregulation of cyclooxygenase-2, Bcl-2, and cell proliferation in the glandular epithelium. Prostate 2004;61:60–72.

[39] Kakehi Y, Segawa T, Wu XX, et al. Down-regulation of macrophage inhibitory cytokine-1/prostate derived factor in benign prostatic hyperplasia. Prostate 2004;59:351–6.

[40] Vykhovanets EV, Resnick MI, Marengo SR. The healthy rat prostate contains high levels of natural killer-like cells and unique subsets of CD4+ helper-inducer T cells: implications for prostatitis. J Urol 2005;173:1004–10.

[41] Kramer G, Mitteregger D, Marberger M. Is benign prostatic hyperplasia (bph) an immune inflammatory disease? Eur Urol 2007;51:1202–16.

[42] Roehrborn CG. Definition of at-risk patients: baseline variables. BJU Int 2006;97(Suppl 2):7–11.

[43] Merendino RA, Salvo F, Saija A, et al. Malondialdehyde in benign prostatic hypertrophy: a useful marker? Mediators Inflamm 2003;12:127–8.

[44] Rohrmann S, De Marzo AM, Smit E, et al. Serum C-reactive protein concentration and lower urinary tract symptoms in older men in the third national health and nutrition examination survey (NHANES III). Prostate 2005;52:43–58.

[45] Castro P, Xia C, Gomez L, et al. Interleukin-8 exression is increased in senescent prostatic epithelial cells and promotes the development of benign prostatic hyperplasia. Prostate 2005;60:153–9.

[46] Penna G, Mondaini N, Amuchastegui S, et al. Seminal plasma cytokines and chemokines in prostate inflammation: interleukin-8 as a predictive biomarker in chronic prostatitis/chronic pelvic pain syndrome and benign prostatic hyperplasia. Eur Urol 2007; 51:524–33.

ELSEVIER
SAUNDERS

Urol Clin N Am 35 (2008) 117–130

UROLOGIC
CLINICS
of North America

Inflammation and Prostate Cancer: A Future Target for Prevention and Therapy?

David Stock, MSc[a,b], Patti A. Groome, PhD[a,b],
D. Robert Siemens, MD, FRCSC[c,d],*

[a]Department of Community Health and Epidemiology, Queen's University,
Abramsky Hall, Arch Street, Kingston, Ontario, Canada K7L 3N6
[b]Division of Cancer Care and Epidemiology, Queen's Cancer Research Institute, Queen's University,
10 Stuart Street, Kingston, Ontario, Canada K7L 3N6
[c]Department of Anatomy and Cell Biology, Queen's University,
Botterell Hall, Room 915, Stuart Street, Kingston, Ontario, Canada K7L 3N6
[d]Department of Urology, Kingston General Hospital, Queen's University, Empire 4, KGH,
76 Stuart St., Kingston, Ontario, Canada, K7L 2V7

Prostate cancer occurs as a consequence of numerous epigenetic and somatic genetic changes, with the subsequent alterations in activation status of a host of oncogenes and tumor suppressor genes. However, no highly penetrant hereditary cancer genes have been consistently identified, despite the important observations of a genetic component to prostate cancer risk. Furthermore, epidemiologic studies, including those investigating dietary and lifestyle differences and cancer risk, highly suggest that suffering from prostate cancer is not simply a result of aging. The discrepancy between prevalence rates of Asia and the Western world, and the finding that Japanese men develop susceptibility to the disease within one generation of immigrating to westernized countries, indicates an important environmental component to prostate cancer etiology [1,2].

Given its long natural history, prostate cancer has become an ideal model for the clinical and basic science study of these environmental contributions to the neoplastic process in several distinct physiologic phases: tumor initiation, progression, invasion, and metastasis. Tumor initiation is attributed to the clonal dominance of cells that undergo genetic mutation and epigenetic changes, resulting in unchecked proliferation [3,4]. Mechanisms that regulate epigenetic processes, thereby altering gene expression without directly modifying the host's genome, are highly sensitive to extrinsic factors, such as diet and related oxidative stress [5]. Stromal facilitation contributes to tumor progression [6], which coupled with insufficient innate tumor suppression and lack of timely clinical intervention, culminates in local invasion and metastasis. Since the first described association between inflammatory infiltrates and proliferative epithelial atrophy in the prostate, a growing body of histopathologic, molecular, and epidemiologic evidence indicates that inflammation plays a key role in the promotion of these neoplastic processes [7–9]. Multiple investigators have demonstrated that prolonged localization of inflammatory cells and mediators can lead to the degradation of tissue architecture, disrupt homeostatic signaling, and cause genomic instability in premalignant, malignant, and stromal tissues.

The following overview of the link between inflammation and prostate cancer serves as a background for the summary of experimental and epidemiologic evidence implicating the inflammatory condition as a promoter of abnormal proliferation, tumor initiation, progression, and even metastasis. A substantial proportion of this

* Corresponding author. Department of Urology, Kingston General Hospital, Queen's University, Empire 4, KGH, 76 Stuart St., Kingston, Ontario, Canada, K7L 2V7.

E-mail address: siemensr@kgh.kari.net (D.R. Siemens).

0094-0143/08/$ - see front matter © 2008 Elsevier Inc. All rights reserved.
doi:10.1016/j.ucl.2007.09.006

urologic.theclinics.com

article is devoted to the discussion of the recent literature on nonsteroidal anti-inflammatory drugs (NSAIDs) and prostate cancer. Evidence supporting potential chemoprotective, and even therapeutic, effects of these drugs through the attenuation of inflammatory processes and the inhibition of cyclooxygenase (COX)-2 gives further credence to the association between inflammation and prostate cancer, and sets the stage for consideration of their usefulness in the prevention and management of this disease.

Inflammation and prostate cancer

A positive association between prostatic inflammation and onset of cancer has been reported in a handful of population studies [8]. Dennis and colleagues [10] summarize corresponding research with a meta-analysis, including all relevant cohort and case-controlled studies published between 1966 and 2000. Out of all included studies (11 case-controlled designs) only three displayed significant findings, though all in the direction of a positive association. The investigators reported an overall increased likelihood of prostate cancer among those with prostatitis. The strength of the association is potentially undermined because of the possibility of a detection bias, given the association between elevated prostate-specific antigen (PSA) and prostatic inflammation [11]. In addition, exposure classification for all but two of the comprising studies was based on self-report. Conversely, the association could have also been biased toward the null as a result of past asymptomatic or undiagnosed prostatitis among cases, as such conditions are prevalent in developed countries [8]. A subsequent case-controlled study reported an increased likelihood of malignancy among men with acute or chronic bacterial prostatitis [12], bolstering support for the transforming potential of inflammation on prostatic tissue. The investigators claimed that, as a result of the high use of PSA screening, misclassification resulting from undiagnosed prostatic inflammatory conditions was less probable.

It has been estimated that as many as 15% of malignancies diagnosed worldwide can be traced to infections [13]. Viruses can facilitate oncogenic initiation directly through modification of the host genome, yet it is plausible that inflammation associated with chronic infection may contribute to the development of prostate cancer [14]. That chronic infections cause inflammation of the prostate is supported by Sutcliffe and colleagues [15],

who observed substantial increases in PSA concentrations after contraction of sexually transmitted infections in younger men. A recent meta-analysis of 29 case-controlled studies published between 1966 and 2004 reported an overall increased likelihood of prostate cancer among individuals who have had sexually transmitted diseases [16]. Experimental evidence has suggested causative roles of these infections in the etiology of prostate cancer. Moyret-Lalle and colleagues [17] observed human papilloma virus (HPV)-16-specific DNA sequences in prostate tumors, while Dillner and colleagues [18] reported a 2.6-fold greater risk of developing prostate cancer among individuals with HPV-18-specific antibodies relative to controls. An association between HPV infections and prostate cancer is further supported by the above meta-analysis that reported increased odds of the malignancy for individuals who claimed to have had previous infections [16].

Inflammation and carcinogenesis

The hypothesis that inflammation acts as an intermediary between infection (or other physical or chemical noxious stimuli) and oncogenesis, gains credibility in light of how inflammatory mediators interact with affected tissue. Inflammation, the homeostatic response to tissue insult, results in edema and the localization of hematocytes and inflammatory cells, and the sequestering of cytokines, eicosanoids, and other chemical messengers [19]. Though usually transient, this process can become self-perpetuating in cases where antagonizing stimuli persist. Prolonged exposure to factors designed to access and destroy invading pathogens leads to the degradation of tissue architecture, disruption in homeostatic signaling, and genomic instability, culminating in abnormal proliferation and tumor initiation.

Disruption of homeostatic signaling

Cell to cell and cell to extra cellular matrix (ECM) contacts within epithelia are crucial in the governance of proliferation [6,20]. Signaling facilitated by these physical interactions, mediated through membrane spanning proteins, has been observed to convey tumor-suppressive functions. The loss of function of one such protein, E-cadherin, is common in epithelial cancers [21] and its role as an inhibitor of progression to a more aggressive phenotype has been observed in vitro, wherein induced functional loss of this integrin stimulated invasion and migration of prostate cancer cells [22]. The over-abundance of proteolytic enzymes produced during inflammation is known to disrupt epithelial cell to cell and cell to ECM adhesions. Matrix metalloproteinases (MMP), notorious degraders of the ECM, released by stromal cells in response to inflammatory response-derived chemical signaling [9], have recently been attributed with multiple functions, including the direct cleavage of integrin molecules such as E-cadherin [23]. Such disruptions in cell to cell signaling is thought to lead to genomic instability and subsequent oncogenic transformation by effecting loss of control over cytokinesis-regulating pathways, such as those mediated by TP53. In support of this, Radisky and colleagues [24] reported a series of experiments demonstrating that addition of MMP-3 to murine mammary cells caused a shift toward malignancy, attributed to altered gene expression, and the resulting increase in reactive oxygen species.

Oxidative stress

Oxidative stress is a well-documented cause of genomic instability and has been implicated in the promotion of tumourigenesis. Activated phagocytes (and potentially epithelial cells) at the site of inflammation produce elevated levels of the superoxide anion, a precursor to a variety of reactive oxygen and nitrogen species [19]. Additional oxidative stress through the accumulation of free radicals from the metabolism of saturated fats and paucity of dietary antioxidants characteristic of Western culture may serve to further disrupt the cellular oxidative balance and increase the likelihood of oncogenic initiation. Peroxidases particular to neutrophils and eosinophils have been observed to be responsible for the production of reactive nitrogen species in murine models of acute inflammation [25], which has additionally been shown to be a precursor of lipid peroxidation [26]. Constant localized exposure to oxidative stress and mediators of the immune response have been implicated in the development of permanent genetic damage and the activation of proto-oncogenes, such as c-fos and c-jun [27]. In a review of a series of human and animal studies, Kawanishi and Hiraku [28] report examples of bacterial, viral, and parasitic infections, as well as noninfectious chronic inflammatory illnesses, that are suspected risk factors for cancer. In these studies, the investigators were able to consistently identify oxidation products of guanine, including

those known to comprise mutagenic DNA lesions in inflammatory and epithelial cells at the site of inflammation. The investigators concluded that these oxidative alterations of DNA were probable contributors to the development of carcinomas from chronic or repeated inflammation caused by helicobacter pylori, hepatitis C, inflammatory bowel disease, and oral lichen planus, at their respective sites. Though the reviewed body of research did not include inflammation of the prostate, many of the same pathologic processes are present in models of chronic prostatitis.

In a recent case-controlled study, Zhou and colleagues [29] compared levels of oxidative stress in 70 subjects with chronic bacterial prostatitis to that of an equal number of healthy controls. The investigators observed increased levels of molecular byproducts of oxidizing reactions and lower activities of prominent antioxidant enzymes among cases. This supports a higher exposure to oxidative stress among the former group, which could potentially result in mutagenic DNA lesions and ultimately, carcinogenesis.

Further epidemiologic support for the transforming effect of reactive oxygen and nitrogen species in prostate epithelia is found in case-controlled studies examining the allele frequency of genes encoding enzymes that protect against, and repair, oxidative damage. Manganese superoxide dismutase is an antioxidant enzyme accredited with the detoxification of oxygen-free radicals inside the mitochondria and has been observed to suppress proliferation of prostate cancer cells both in vitro and in vivo [30]. A polymorphism for the encoding gene was discovered that consists of a single valine-alanine substitution, thought to affect the enzyme's ability to permeate the mitochondrial membrane. Results from a study nested within the α-tocopherol β-carotene Cancer Prevention Study by Woodson and colleagues [31] imply that men homozygous for the alanine allele had an increased risk of prostate cancer. Two independent case-controlled studies reported increased prostate cancer risk with certain polymorphisms of a gene encoding human oxoguanine glycosylase, an enzyme involved in repair of oxidative DNA lesions [32,33]. An increased risk for men with the Ser362Cys polymorphism was common to both. Evidence that reduced functionality of innate antioxidant mechanisms can increase the likelihood of developing prostate cancer coincides with the idea that sustained, elevated oxidative stress, as encountered in chronic inflammation, is a probable potent carcinogen.

Glutathione-S-transferases (GSTs) are an important family of antioxidant enzymes that, because of their role as detoxifiers of reactive compounds, have been postulated to provide protection against oncogenesis [34]. The enzymes are capable of neutralizing several different forms of potentially damaging reactive products and are basally expressed in normal epithelial cells [35]. However, a recent meta-analysis assessing the association between certain genetic variations of three of the most common GST genes (GSTM1, GSTT1 and GSTP1) and risk of prostate cancer was unable to detect a statistically significant association [36]. The investigators chose studies that compared null and nondeleted genotypes for GSTM1 and GSTT1, and two common polymorphisms for GSTP1. The quantitative synthesis of cases and controls from 11, 10, and 12 studies on GSTM1, GSTT1 and GSTP1, respectively, failed to show significant allelic differences for the GST genes between cases and healthy controls, yet loss of GST functionality is ubiquitous in prostate [8,37]. The nearly unanimous down-regulation of GSTP1 in high-grade intraepithelial neoplasia (HGPIN) and carcinomas imply a "caretaker" role, described by Kinzler and Vogelstein [38] as a gene whose inactivation facilitates genomic instability, resulting tumor initiation.

This loss of function has been attributed to the somatic silencing of GST genes, corroborated by Lin and colleagues [39], who observed that 95% of assessed prostatectomy and lymph node dissection samples exhibited hypermethylation of distinct sequences in the promoter region of GSTP1. Parsons and colleagues [35] observed that GSTP1, the most widely studied of the GST enzymes within the human prostate, is highly expressed in normal prostate epithelium, while GSTPA1 is not. The investigators noted that regions of focal prostatic glandular atrophy, potential precursors to HGPIN, display elevated GSTP1 and GSTPA1 activity, while both are down-regulated in HGPIN and adenocarcinomas. The evidence behind such a prominent group of antioxidant enzymes having this caretaker role in prostate tumourigenesis further upholds the hypothesis of inflammation-induced carcinogenesis via disruption of oxidative balance.

Inflammation and progression

Recent syntheses of the literature depict chronic or recurrent inflammatory environments wherein persistent leukocyte recruitment and activation can stimulate tumor progression through the overproduction of various inflammatory mediators [7,9,40,41]. Localization of leukocytes to the tumor environment has been recognized for many years, though the implications of this were, for a long time, largely ignored [9,41]. More recently, tumor associated macrophage (TAM) density has been positively correlated with poor clinical outcome at multiple sites [42], yet findings for some cancer types were inconsistent. One of the studies supporting this association reported that increased TAM density was associated with shorter survival time for patients with prostate carcinomas [43]. In addition to the increased production of reactive oxygen and nitrogen species associated with the metabolism of saturated fats, another facet through which the westernized diet may promote prostate cancer via inflammatory processes is through its relatively high content of heterocyclic amines produced from the cooking of meat at high temperatures. Among the proposed mechanisms by which their accumulation contributes to initiation and progression, animal models have indicated selective sequestering of macrophages within the prostate upon exposure to these compounds [44]. The following is a summary of some key inflammatory mediators produced by activated leukocytes and stromal cells that are likely contributors to the progression to a more aggressive tumor phenotype.

Tumor associated macrophages

Inflammatory factors produced by TAMs directly, through paracrine interaction with other cells or by liberation from the breakdown of stromal tissue, contribute to malignancy by multiple processes, three of the most significant being resistance to apoptosis, induction of proliferation, and angiogenesis [9,45]. Originating from circulating monocytes, TAMs are a major constituent of the leukocytes that infiltrate the tumor microenvironment [45]. TAM function is modified by exposure to various cytokines and has been observed to confer both tumor-suppressing and promoting activity. Two studies exposing macrophages to interleukin (IL)-12, one directly and the other via injection with a vector containing the IL-12 gene, noted a resulting tumouricidal behavior of TAMs, both in vitro and in vivo, toward chemically induced tumors [46,47].

Other research has implicated TAMs as promoters of tumor progression because of the production of proangiogenic growth factors, cytokines, and proteases [9,40,45]. Torisu and colleagues [48], observed that the up-regulation of vascular endothelial growth factor (VEGF), a strong promoter of angiogenesis, corresponded with increased production of proinflammatory cytokines produced by activated macrophages. The investigators noted that degree of macrophage infiltration was correlated with microvessel density and depth of tumor invasion in melanomas, directly implicating TAMs in the promotion of angiogenesis and tumor progression. Positive correlations between TAM infiltration of the tumor environment, VEGF levels, and microvessel density have also been observed in human breast and oral cancers [49,50]. That TAMs can behave as both tumor suppressors and promoters is consistent with the current concept of a tumor microenvironment that enlists host immune response mechanisms to enhance malignant progression [45,51]. A key component of this is the reprogramming of TAMs and other immune cells through chronic or recurrent exposure to soluble mediators of inflammation.

Soluble inflammatory mediators

Chemokines, originally identified as directors of leukocyte migration [52], provide another example of how inflammation-related host systems might promote tumor progression. These soluble mediators have been attributed with a number of homeostatic roles, including mediation of the infiltration and activation of leukocytes during the inflammatory response [52]. Altered chemokine receptor expression has been observed in neoplastic tissue, particularly near tumor and host tissue borders [40]. Evidence for inflammation-associated chemokines as potentiators of malignancy, specific to prostate cancer, is found in recent studies reporting elevated expression of them and their receptors in human prostate cancer cell lines. Increased expression of members of the CXC family of chemokines, implicated in the promotion of angiogenesis, was found to be correlated with invasiveness of prostate cancer cell lines [53]. This was associated with the cytoplasmic relocalization of corresponding CXC receptors from the cell surface. Murphy and colleagues [54] reported a correlation between increased expression of another member of the CXC chemokine family, IL-8, its receptors, and high-grade disease in human biopsies. Recently, Vaday and colleagues [55] discovered the expression of CCL5 and its receptor, CCR5, in human prostate cancer cells, a chemokine known to

stimulate cell migration in breast cancer and one that has been correlated with the progression of other malignant diseases. In proof of a similar aggressiveness-enhancing effect in prostate cancer, the investigators reported that incubation with exogenous CCL5 stimulated proliferation and increased invasiveness of prostate cancer cells. Cytokines, other soluble mediators of inflammation, have been implicated in the signaling of malignant progression. A key proinflammatory cytokine, tumor necrosis factor-alpha (TNF-α), has demonstrated tumor-promoting behavior at multiple cancer sites [56].

TNF-α is regulated by the proteolytic activity of stromal metalloproteinases that liberate it from membranes of somatic cells [40] and is produced by TAMs directly [9]. Selective blockade of TNF-α and TNF-α receptor expression has resulted in resistance to chemically induced epidermal [57] and hepatic [58] cancers, indicating an important role of TNF-α in tumourigenesis at these, and perhaps other sites. Pikarsky and colleagues [59] used Mdr2 knockout mice, artificially provoking inflammation-derived carcinogenesis, to elucidate mediators involved in this process. The researchers discovered that suppression of nuclear transcription factor (NF)-κB through inhibition of TNF-α resulted in apoptosis of transformed hepatocytes and the arrest of further progression to carcinogenesis. In addition, it was observed that TNF-α at the site of inflammation was not hepatocyte-derived, and concentrations of the cytokine were five-fold in Mdr2 knockout mice relative to wild types, implicating inflammatory or other parenchymal cells as the source. Recently, Huerta-Yepez and colleagues [60] presented evidence of TNF-α having a role in conveying resistance to Fas-induced apoptosis through a similar pathway involving NF-κB in human prostate cancer cells.

NF-κB, known as a master inflammatory transcriptional regulator, has been shown to be activated by reactive oxygen species and various other carcinogens, in addition to pro-inflammatory chemokines and cytokines such as TNF-α [19,45]. It is a potentially multi-faceted instigator of progression to more aggressive phenotypes because of its regulation of gene products that have been observed to be involved in mediating resistance to apoptosis, insensitivity to growth inhibition, tissue invasion, immortalization, and angiogenesis [45]. NF-κB is constitutively active in many tumor cell lines, including transformed androgen-independent PC-3 and DU-145 prostate cells [61], though not in normal epithelial tissue.

Kukreja and colleagues [62] report findings that implicate NF-κB activity in the increased expression of a particular chemokine receptor, CXCR4, that was observed to confer heightened invasiveness in the former of these cell lineages. Recently, Yemelyanov and colleagues [63], were able to induce apoptosis and inhibit proliferation and invasive activity in human androgen-independent prostate carcinoma cell lines using a novel NF-κB inhibitor. The investigators noted that inactivation of NF-κB coincided with reduced production of VEGF from both cell lines, supporting the transcription factor's positive regulation of angiogenesis. Because of its low-specificity for activation and multifarious transcriptional regulation of genes that serve to promote survival and proliferation, NF-κB has been regarded as an overall mediator of the stress response [64]. The idea of inflammation as a predominant stressor of the tumor microenvironment portrays the NF-κB pathway as a key enabler of aggressive tumor characteristics.

Inflammation and metastatic potential

The up-regulation of protease activity has been implicated in invasion and metastasis in addition to oncogenesis. In vitro evidence has shown that interaction between tumor and stromal cells induce phenotypes conducive to invasion through local barriers and metastasis [65]. More specific support for a role of these proteases in invasion is reported by Bair and colleagues [66], who observed that up-regulation of MT1-MMP in prostate cancer cells caused selective degradation of the basement membrane and associated membrane transmigration at cleavage sites. Up-regulation of genes encoding MMPs and other membrane degrading enzymes have additionally been found in prostate tumor cells at distal locations in mice [67,68], implicating a role in metastasis. That increased MMP expression has been associated with elevated levels of reactive oxygen and nitrogen species [69,70] provides a possible link between oxidative stress produced by mediators of inflammation, the migration of tumor cells from the microenvironment, and increased invasive potential characteristic of metastasis.

Nonsteroidal anti-inflammatory drugs as chemoprotective agents

NSAIDs, among the most widely used medications, are endowed with analgesic, antipyretic, and anti-inflammatory actions. Observations that NSAIDs are able to block neutrophil and macrophage accumulation, and repress other crucial inflammatory processes [71], solidify their reputation as effective anti-inflammatory agents. These properties are predominantly, though not exclusively, attributed to their inhibition of COX-2, an enzyme that catalyzes the rate-limiting step in prostaglandin and thromboxane production. Evidence for the now widely-accepted notion that COX-2 blockade is responsible for the anti-inflammatory properties of NSAIDs stems from animal studies that demonstrated inflammation-associated edema and analgesia correspond to elevated levels of prostaglandin E2 [72]. These symptoms were attenuated after exposure to COX-2 inhibitors.

Attenuation of inflammation

The previously discussed evidence indicating a causative relationship between inflammation and malignancy makes the ability to suppress inflammatory symptoms enticing in the elucidation of anti-cancer agents. It is this function that has made these medications popular targets in the search for chemopreventative agents [73], supported by the recognition of inflammatory disorders as risk factors for cancer [19]. Their observed inhibition of COX further strengthens this hypothesis and provides a corresponding mechanistic framework. Fig. 1 provides an overview of inflammation-derived mechanisms that facilitate tumor initiation and progression and depicts NSAIDs as potential inhibitors of these processes.

COX-2, up-regulated during the inflammatory response, is thought to be inducible by a number of proinflammatory cytokines, including TNF-α [74,75]. An example of this relationship in the prostate was presented by Subbarayan and colleagues [76], who found that TNF-α could induce COX-2 expression in both normal prostate and androgen-unresponsive prostate cancer cells. The investigators confirmed that up-regulation of COX-2 was related to increases in cellular levels of prostaglandins. COX-2 expression has been suggested to be dependent on inflammatory cytokine/NF-κB pathways in prostate cancer [77] and other normal cell types [78–80], supporting a possible positive feedback between carcinogenic inflammatory mediators and prostaglandin production. Support for the relationship between chronic inflammation and the up-regulation of

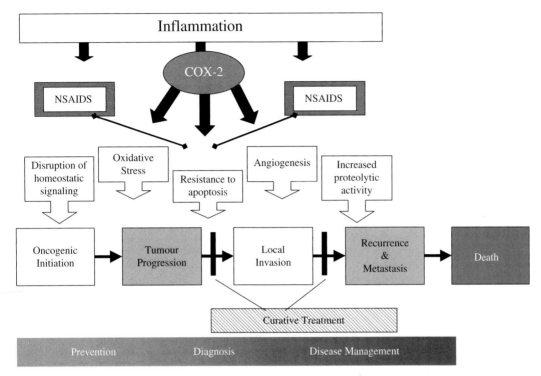

Fig. 1. Contribution of inflammation in the initiation and progression of neoplastic disease and the possible roles of anti-inflammatory medications as therapy. Summary of the potential carcinogenic effects of inflammation over preclinical and clinical phases of the natural history of prostate cancer. NSAIDs, largely through the inhibition COX-2, attenuate inflammatory processes that promote tumor initiation and progression.

COX-2 in the prostate can be observed in series of experiments by Wang and colleagues [81]. The investigators found that foci of chronic inflammation within human samples of benign prostate hyperplasia were associated with accumulation of inflammatory cells. Moderate to high permeation of these cells, particularly T-lymphocytes and macrophages, were highly correlated with positive staining for COX-2. Though the above provides compelling evidence for a potentially protective action against initiation and progression of prostate cancer through the attenuation of inflammation, more direct means by which the up-regulation of COX-2 promotes these processes have been demonstrated.

Inhibition of COX-2

Genetic variation of COX-2 has been associated with differential prostate cancer risk. In their examination of 16 single nucleotide polymorphisms (SNPs), Shahedi and colleagues discovered a significant difference in expression between 1,378 prostate cancer patients and 782 controls at two COX-2 loci. These findings could support a role of COX-2 in the development of prostate cancer if one or both of these SNPs were to confer heightened enzyme activity. The conversion of arachidonic acid into prostaglandins by COX-2 liberates free radicals [27], suggesting a direct oxidizing, and therefore oncogenic, effect of elevated COX-2 activity. Recently, COX-2 inhibitors have been associated with reduced DNA damage in human mucosal cells after exposure to reactive oxygen species [82]. Such findings are indicative of a contributory role in oncogenic transformation and, by the same token, a potential protective effect of NSAIDs on tumor initiation.

Superficial evidence for COX-2 as a promoter of prostatic tumor progression is presented in studies reporting increased expression of the enzyme in human prostate cancer tissue samples [83–88], though at least one such study has reported to the contrary [89]. In addition, Cohen and colleagues [90] determined that COX-2 expression was an independent predictor of disease progression from a multivariate analysis of samples from 60 prostate cancer patients following radical prostatectomy. The potential benefit of COX-2 inhibition in prostate cancer management stems from the enzyme's apparent tumourigenic properties, more specifically its roles in proliferation, angiogenesis, and resistance to apoptosis.

The idea of COX-2 as a promoter of proliferation in prostate cancer is solidified by literature consistently showing that increased expression of the enzyme is correlated with tumor progression. During their in vivo investigation of the effects of COX-2 inhibition on tumor proliferation, Liu and colleagues [91] observed that mice inoculated with human prostate cancer cells produced tumors of markedly reduced surface area when treated with a selective NSAIDs. In a related study, increased prostaglandin E2 production, corresponding with up-regulation of COX-2, was found to induce prostate intraepithelial neoplasia cell growth in vitro [92]. In addition, the investigators were able to stimulate this behavior using IL-6, a notorious proinflammatory cytokine, and inhibit it with selective NSAID treatment. In a second in vitro study, COX-2 blockade by both COX-1 and COX-2-specific inhibitors in DU145, LnCaP, and PC3 prostate cancer cells corresponded with reduced growth in all three lineages [93]. Focusing on the proliferative effects of COX-2, Fujita and colleagues [94] reported that gene amplification of the enzyme in LnCaP cells corresponded with augmented proliferation in vitro and faster growing tumors upon incubation into severe combined immunodeficiency disease mice. The investigators noted that VEGF expression in LnCaP cells with artificially up-regulated COX-2 was significantly higher than in normal cells, and speculated that the larger tumors may be a result of COX-2-induced angiogenesis.

A recent study investigating the correlation between expression levels of COX-2 and VEGF within nonsmall cell lung cancer tumors resected from 60 lung cancer patients, observed a significant increase in VEGF mRNA in samples with higher concentrations of COX-2 gene transcripts [95]. Researchers additionally reported a significant, direct correlation between increased VEGF mRNA and the extent of microvascularization in excised tissue. From follow-up of these patients, investigators discovered a significant inverse trend relating detected concentrations of COX-2 mRNA with patient survival. A correlation

between the up-regulation of COX-2 in response to hypoxia and resulting increased VEGF expression have also been demonstrated in prostate cancer cell lines [96]. Strong support for COX-2 mediated angiogenesis within an inflammatory microenvironment is found in the recent work of Wang and colleagues [83]. The investigators discovered that COX-2 expression, elevated around foci of inflammation, was significantly correlated with increased microvessel density.

The induction of COX-2 has additionally been linked to the blockade of apoptosis. Though this has shown to be mediated through Bcl-2 and Akt signaling [97], the complete delineation of this antiapoptotic effect is arguably elusive. Liu and colleagues [98] studied the tumourigenic potential of COX-2 over-expression in transgenic mice and observed that up-regulation of the enzyme coincided with elevated levels of the anti-apoptotic protein, Bcl-2. In a related study, treatment of prostate cancer cells (LNCaP) with a selective COX-2 inhibitor was shown to similarly reduce Bcl-2 expression. This was associated with chromosomal degradation and a subsequent increase in apoptosis [99]. Dandekar and Lokeshwar [100] observed that phosphorylation (and subsequent activation) of Akt, a protein involved in apoptosis resistance, was decreased in COX-2 depleted prostate cancer cells relative to controls. The investigators concluded that apoptosis in COX-2 deficient PC-3 mL cells occurred eight times more frequently, while microvessel density was three times lower compared with cells expressing high levels of COX-2, providing additional support for a promoting role of COX-2 in both angiogenesis and overall tumor progression.

Further evidence that induced COX-2 conveys apoptotic resistance to prostate tumors comes from Huh and colleagues [101], who demonstrated that sanguinarine-induced apoptosis of LNCaP cells, constitutively low COX-2 producers, was decreased in cell variants with amplified COX-2 genes. The investigators observed that the apoptotic effect of sanguinarine was accompanied with increased nitric oxide (NO) production, that apoptosis could be attenuated with a NO synthase inhibitor, and that COX-2 transfection of LNCaP cells corresponded to lower NO formation. This indicates that COX-2-mediated apoptotic resistance was attributed, at least in part, to the inhibition of NO production. The antiapoptotic effects of COX-2 have also been postulated to be mediated through suppression of TP53 [99,102].

There have been indications that COX-2 may also contribute to invasive potential, shown to be largely a factor of net proteolytic activity, of a given tumor cell. Similarly, the abundance of active proteases, particularly MMPs, may also have bearing on metastatic propensity. Assessing the effect of prostaglandin synthesis on the invasiveness of prostate tumor cells, Attiga and colleagues [103] observed that DU-145 cell invasion through a solubilized basement membrane preparation was reduced after treatment with both ibuprophen and a selective COX-2 inhibitor, in comparison with controls, the latter producing the effect in a dose-dependent manner. Using electrophoretic techniques, investigators noted that this attenuated invasiveness was associated with a reduction in the concentration of pro-MMP-2 and MMP-2 secreted into the culture medium. That invasive behavior could be reestablished by incubation with prostaglandin E2, the immediate downstream product of the enzyme, indicates that the anti-invasive effect of NSAID treatment was COX-2 dependent.

NSAIDs and risk of prostate cancer

There have been numerous epidemiologic studies investigating the association between NSAID use and risk of cancer, particularly at colorectal, breast, and prostatic sites. In their review and synthesis of 91 relevant epidemiologic studies, Harris and colleagues [104] found a significant exponential decrease in cancer risk with heavier NSAID regimens for 7 out of 10 cancer types. The researchers reported a significantly declining risk of prostate cancer with increasing number of pills taken per week. Some of the most dramatic evidence supporting reduced prostate cancer risk with NSAID use was presented by Roberts and colleagues [105] and Nelson and Harris [106], who found overall reductions in likelihood of disease of 55% and 66%, respectively, for users of these medications.

To ascertain whether epidemiologic evidence was reflective of experimental findings suggestive of a protective capacity of these drugs, Mahmud and colleagues [107] conducted a meta-analysis of relevant studies published before 2003. The combination of the nine studies that investigated aspirin usage alone demonstrated reduced odds of prostate cancer. The amalgamation of results from studies investigating total NSAID use or nonacetylsalicylic acid NSAIDs yielded risk estimates denoting a similar trend, but were not statistically significant. The instability of the risk estimates is likely accounted for, at least in part, by the heterogeneity of the comprising data: parameters such as duration and dosage were measured differently across the included studies.

Out of the relevant studies published after the above meta-analysis, one has produced results which, though suggestive of a possible protective effect, are not statistically significant [108], while two recent case-controlled studies have achieved results that are contradictory [109,110]. It is important to note, however, that exposure classification for the latter two case-controlled studies are suspect, as it was based on retrospective self-reported aspirin use. As aspirin is one of the most easily accessible and widely consumed of the nonprescription NSAIDs, there may be some potential for misclassification and recall bias. Five additional studies upheld a protective effect of NSAIDs [108,111–114]. The largest (70,144 men included in the analysis) and most recent of these reported that a long duration and regular use of NSAIDs (at least 30 pills per month for 5 years) was associated with a decreased risk of prostate cancer [114].

NSAIDs and prostate cancer outcomes

Epidemiologic research assessing the effect of NSAIDs on the progression of prostate cancer is sparse. Mahmud and colleagues [113], in corroboration with the authors' own unpublished results, found that there was a reduced likelihood of highly aggressive disease (total Gleason score of 8 or higher) at diagnosis for NSAID users. While there have been a handful of pilot and phase II clinical trials looking at the effects of COX-2 inhibitors on advanced stage colon and breast cancers [97], there have only been two groups that have published comparable studies on prostate cancer outcomes. Both, investigating celecoxib in the prevention of biochemical failure, found that selective COX-2 inhibition was able to suppress the rate of PSA increase in prostate cancer patients after curative treatment. A pilot study on the effect of selective COX-2 inhibitors on the doubling time of PSA levels after biochemical failure found that 8 of the 12 subjects experienced a significant attenuation of increasing PSA concentration [115]. In the subsequent phase II randomized trial, 36 out of 40 subjects showed a drop in the rate of PSA increase [116], while 8 of these subjects responded with stabilization of PSA levels and 11 demonstrated absolute decreases in PSA concentrations. Smith and colleagues [117] reported on the effects of celecoxib in the prevention of metastatic progression in men with recurrent disease. Fifteen out of 38 men randomly assigned to receive celecoxib, compared with the 8 out of 40 who received a placebo, achieved a 200% increase in PSA doubling time without detection of metastasis. Men taking celecoxib also demonstrated a slightly slower rate of PSA increase. Though this may indicate some benefit of NSAIDs to patients with advanced disease, the implications of these findings are uncertain. Furthermore, the latter-most study was terminated early because of discovery of potential cardiac side effects of selective-COX-2 inhibitors. Though PSA metrics are of proven prognostic importance, the biologic implication of such changes in PSA concentrations have yet to be fully delineated.

Summary

Though there is strong evidence implicating individual inflammatory mediators and byproducts as promoters of tumor initiation and disease progression, the overall impact of inflammation on prostate cancer is complex and continues to be elusive. It is perhaps possible that inflammation is merely symptomatic of a tissue environment more susceptible to malignancy, given the activation or silencing of other related factors, rather than a direct intermediary between extrinsic insult and prostate cancer. However, until prostate carcinogenesis is better understood, the potential for interventions that successfully inhibit inflammatory processes cannot be ignored. Though their efficacy in the prevention of adverse disease outcomes is unclear, the literature has consistently demonstrated reduced cancer risk, at the prostate and other sites, for people using NSAIDs. The usefulness of interventions such as NSAIDs in prostate cancer management can only be substantiated by larger cohort studies and clinical trials that focus on endpoints that are established indicators of disease invasiveness.

References

[1] Crawford ED. Epidemiology of prostate cancer. Urology 2003;62(6 Suppl 1):3–12.
[2] Pu YS, Chiang HS, Lin CC, et al. Changing trends of prostate cancer in Asia. Aging Male 2004;7(2):120–32.
[3] Nowell PC. Mechanisms of tumor progression. Cancer Res 1986;46(5):2203–7.
[4] Kerbel RS, Waghorne C, Korczak B, et al. Clonal dominance of primary tumours by metastatic cells: genetic analysis and biological implications. Cancer Surv 1988;7(4):597–629.
[5] Dobosy JR, Roberts JL, Fu VX, et al. The expanding role of epigenetics in the development, diagnosis and treatment of prostate cancer and benign prostatic hyperplasia. J Urol 2007;177(3):822–31.
[6] Liotta LA, Kohn EC. The microenvironment of the tumour-host interface. Nature 2001;411(6835):375–9.
[7] Balkwill F, Charles KA, Mantovani A. Smoldering and polarized inflammation in the initiation and promotion of malignant disease. Cancer Cell 2005;7(3):211–7.
[8] Nelson WG, De Marzo AM, DeWeese TL, et al. The role of inflammation in the pathogenesis of prostate cancer. J Urol 2004;172(5 Pt 2):S6–11.
[9] Pollard JW. Tumour-educated macrophages promote tumour progression and metastasis. Nat Rev Cancer 2004;4(1):71–8.
[10] Dennis LK, Lynch CF, Torner JC. Epidemiologic association between prostatitis and prostate cancer. Urology 2002;60(1):78–83.
[11] Kawakami J, Siemens DR, Nickel JC. Prostatitis and prostate cancer: implications for prostate cancer screening. Urology 2004;64(6):1075–80.
[12] Roberts RO, Bergstralh EJ, Bass SE, et al. Prostatitis as a risk factor for prostate cancer. Epidemiology 2004;15(1):93–9.
[13] Coussens LM, Werb Z. Inflammation and cancer. Nature 2002;420(6917):860–7.
[14] Ohshima H, Tatemichi M, Sawa T. Chemical basis of inflammation-induced carcinogenesis. Arch Biochem Biophys 2003;417(1):3–11.
[15] Sutcliffe S, Zenilman JM, Ghanem KG, et al. Sexually transmitted infections and prostatic inflammation/cell damage as measured by serum prostate specific antigen concentration. J Urol 2006;175(5):1937–42.
[16] Taylor ML, Mainous AG III, Wells BJ. Prostate cancer and sexually transmitted diseases: a meta-analysis. Fam Med 2005;37(7):506–12.
[17] Moyret-Lalle C, Marcais C, Jacquemier J, et al. Ras, p53 and HPV status in benign and malignant prostate tumors. Int J Cancer 1995;64(2):124–9.
[18] Dillner J, Knekt P, Boman J, et al. Sero-epidemiological association between human-papillomavirus infection and risk of prostate cancer. Int J Cancer 1998;75(4):564–7.
[19] Ohshima H, Tazawa H, Sylla BS, et al. Prevention of human cancer by modulation of chronic inflammatory processes. Mutat Res 2005;591(1-2):110–22.
[20] Bissell MJ, Radisky D. Putting tumours in context. Nat Rev Cancer 2001;1(1):46–54.
[21] Christofori G, Semb H. The role of the cell-adhesion molecule E-cadherin as a tumour-suppressor gene. Trends Biochem Sci 1999;24(2):73–6.

[22] Chunthapong J, Seftor EA, Khalkhali-Ellis Z, et al. Dual roles of E-cadherin in prostate cancer invasion. J Cell Biochem 2004;91(4):649–61.

[23] Radisky DC, Bissell MJ. Matrix metalloproteinase-induced genomic instability. Curr Opin Genet Dev 2006;16(1):45–50.

[24] Radisky DC, Levy DD, Littlepage LE, et al. Rac1b and reactive oxygen species mediate MMP-3-induced EMT and genomic instability. Nature 2005;436(7047):123–7.

[25] Zhang R, Brennan ML, Shen Z, et al. Myeloperoxidase functions as a major enzymatic catalyst for initiation of lipid peroxidation at sites of inflammation. J Biol Chem 2002;277(48):46116–22.

[26] Brennan ML, Wu W, Fu X, et al. A tale of two controversies: defining both the role of peroxidases in nitrotyrosine formation in vivo using eosinophil peroxidase and myeloperoxidase-deficient mice, and the nature of peroxidase-generated reactive nitrogen species. J Biol Chem 2002;277(20):17415–27.

[27] Pathak SK, Sharma RA, Steward WP, et al. Oxidative stress and cyclooxygenase activity in prostate carcinogenesis: targets for chemopreventive strategies. Eur J Cancer 2005;41(1):61–70.

[28] Kawanishi S, Hiraku Y. Oxidative and nitrative DNA damage as biomarker for carcinogenesis with special reference to inflammation. Antioxid Redox Signal 2006;8(5–6):1047–58.

[29] Zhou JF, Xiao WQ, Zheng YC, et al. Increased oxidative stress and oxidative damage associated with chronic bacterial prostatitis. Asian J Androl 2006;8(3):317–23.

[30] Li N, Oberley TD, Oberley LW, et al. Overexpression of manganese superoxide dismutase in DU145 human prostate carcinoma cells has multiple effects on cell phenotype. Prostate 1998;35(3):221–33.

[31] Woodson K, Tangrea JA, Lehman TA, et al. Manganese superoxide dismutase (MnSOD) polymorphism, alpha-tocopherol supplementation and prostate cancer risk in the alpha-tocopherol, beta-carotene cancer prevention study (Finland). Cancer Causes Control 2003;14(6):513–8.

[32] Xu J, Zheng SL, Turner A, et al. Associations between hOGG1 sequence variants and prostate cancer susceptibility. Cancer Res 2002;62(8):2253–7.

[33] Chen L, Elahi A, Pow-Sang J, et al. Association between polymorphism of human oxoguanine glycosylase 1 and risk of prostate cancer. J Urol 2003;170(6 Pt 1):2471–4.

[34] Hayes JD, Pulford DJ. The glutathione S-transferase supergene family: regulation of GST and the contribution of the isoenzymes to cancer chemoprotection and drug resistance. Crit Rev Biochem Mol Biol 1995;30(6):445–600.

[35] Parsons JK, Nelson CP, Gage WR, et al. GSTA1 expression in normal, preneoplastic, and neoplastic human prostate tissue. Prostate 2001;49(1):30–7.

[36] Ntais C, Polycarpou A, Ioannidis JP. Association of GSTM1, GSTT1, and GSTP1 gene polymorphisms with the risk of prostate cancer: a meta-analysis. Cancer Epidemiol Biomarkers Prev 2005;14(1):176–81.

[37] De Marzo AM, Meeker AK, Zha S, et al. Human prostate cancer precursors and pathobiology. Urology 2003;62(5 Suppl 1):55–62.

[38] Kinzler KW, Vogelstein B. Cancer-susceptibility genes. Gatekeepers and caretakers. Nature 1997;386(6627):761–3.

[39] Lin X, Tascilar M, Lee WH, et al. GSTP1 CpG island hypermethylation is responsible for the absence of GSTP1 expression in human prostate cancer cells. Am J Pathol 2001;159(5):1815–26.

[40] Robinson SC, Coussens LM. Soluble mediators of inflammation during tumor development. Advances in cancer research 2005;93:159–87.

[41] Rollins BJ. Inflammatory chemokines in cancer growth and progression. Eur J Cancer 2006;42(6):760–7.

[42] Bingle L, Brown NJ, Lewis CE. The role of tumour-associated macrophages in tumour progression: implications for new anticancer therapies. J Pathol 2002;196(3):254–65.

[43] Lissbrant IF, Stattin P, Wikstrom P, et al. Tumor associated macrophages in human prostate cancer: relation to clinicopathological variables and survival. Int J Oncol 2000;17(3):445–51.

[44] Nakai Y, Nelson WG, De Marzo AM. The dietary charred meat carcinogen 2-amino-1-methyl-6-phenylimidazo [4,5-b] pyridine acts as both a tumor initiator and promoter in the rat ventral prostate. Cancer Res 2007;67(3):1378–84.

[45] Mantovani A, Schioppa T, Porta C, et al. Role of tumor-associated macrophages in tumor progression and invasion. Cancer Metastasis Rev 2006;25(3):315–22.

[46] Satoh T, Saika T, Ebara S, et al. Macrophages transduced with an adenoviral vector expressing interleukin 12 suppress tumor growth and metastasis in a preclinical metastatic prostate cancer model. Cancer Res 2003;63(22):7853–60.

[47] Tsung K, Dolan JP, Tsung YL, et al. Macrophages as effector cells in interleukin 12-induced T cell-dependent tumor rejection. Cancer Res 2002;62(17):5069–75.

[48] Torisu H, Ono M, Kiryu H, et al. Macrophage infiltration correlates with tumor stage and angiogenesis in human malignant melanoma: possible involvement of TNF-alpha and IL-1alpha. Int J Cancer 2000;85(2):182–8.

[49] Tsutsui S, Yasuda K, Suzuki K, et al. Macrophage infiltration and its prognostic implications in breast cancer: the relationship with VEGF expression and microvessel density. Oncol Rep 2005;14(2):425–31.

[50] Li C, Shintani S, Terakado N, et al. Infiltration of tumor-associated macrophages in human oral

squamous cell carcinoma. Oncol Rep 2002;9(6): 1219–23.

[51] Whiteside TL. Immune suppression in cancer: effects on immune cells, mechanisms and future therapeutic intervention. Semin Cancer Biol 2006; 16(1):3–15.

[52] Le Y, Zhou Y, Iribarren P, et al. Chemokines and chemokine receptors: their manifold roles in homeostasis and disease. Cell Mol Immunol 2004; 1(2):95–104.

[53] Engl T, Relja B, Blumenberg C, et al. Prostate tumor CXC-chemokine profile correlates with cell adhesion to endothelium and extracellular matrix. Life Sci 2006;78(16):1784–93.

[54] Murphy C, McGurk M, Pettigrew J, et al. Nonapical and cytoplasmic expression of interleukin-8, CXCR1, and CXCR2 correlates with cell proliferation and microvessel density in prostate cancer. Clin Cancer Res 2005;11(11):4117–27.

[55] Vaday GG, Peehl DM, Kadam PA, et al. Expression of CCL5 (RANTES) and CCR5 in prostate cancer. Prostate 2006;66(2):124–34.

[56] Balkwill F. TNF-alpha in promotion and progression of cancer. Cancer Metastasis Rev 2006;25(3): 409–16.

[57] Moore RJ, Owens DM, Stamp G, et al. Mice deficient in tumor necrosis factor-alpha are resistant to skin carcinogenesis. Nat Med 1999;5(7):828–31.

[58] Knight B, Yeoh GC, Husk KL, et al. Impaired preneoplastic changes and liver tumor formation in tumor necrosis factor receptor type 1 knockout mice. J Exp Med 2000;192(12):1809–18.

[59] Pikarsky E, Porat RM, Stein I, et al. NF-kappaB functions as a tumour promoter in inflammation-associated cancer. Nature 2004;431(7007):461–6.

[60] Huerta-Yepez S, Vega M, Garban H, et al. Involvement of the TNF-alpha autocrine-paracrine loop, via NF-kappaB and YY1, in the regulation of tumor cell resistance to Fas-induced apoptosis. Clin Immunol 2006;120(3):297–309.

[61] Palayoor ST, Youmell MY, Calderwood SK, et al. Constitutive activation of IkappaB kinase alpha and NF-kappaB in prostate cancer cells is inhibited by ibuprofen. Oncogene 1999;18(51):7389–94.

[62] Kukreja P, Adel-Mageed AB, Mondal D, et al. Up-regulation of CXCR4 expression in PC-3 cells by stromal-derived factor-1alpha (CXCL12) increases endothelial adhesion and transendothelial migration: role of MEK/ERK signaling pathway-dependent NF-kappaB activation. Cancer Res 2005; 65(21):9891–8.

[63] Yemelyanov A, Gasparian A, Lindholm P, et al. Effects of IKK inhibitor PS1145 on NF-kappaB function, proliferation, apoptosis and invasion activity in prostate carcinoma cells. Oncogene 2006; 25(3):387–98.

[64] Pahl HL. Activators and target genes of Rel/NF-kappaB transcription factors. Oncogene 1999; 18(49):6853–66.

[65] Kaminski A, Hahne JC, Haddouti el-M, et al. Tumour-stroma interactions between metastatic prostate cancer cells and fibroblasts. Int J Mol Med 2006;18(5):941–50.

[66] Bair EL, Chen ML, McDaniel K, et al. Membrane type 1 matrix metalloprotease cleaves laminin-10 and promotes prostate cancer cell migration. Neoplasia 2005;7(4):380–9.

[67] Aalinkeel R, Nair MP, Sufrin G, et al. Gene expression of angiogenic factors correlates with metastatic potential of prostate cancer cells. Cancer Res 2004;64(15):5311–21.

[68] Chu JH, Sun ZY, Meng XL, et al. Differential metastasis-associated gene analysis of prostate carcinoma cells derived from primary tumor and spontaneous lymphatic metastasis in nude mice with orthotopic implantation of PC-3M cells. Cancer Lett 2006;233(1):79–88.

[69] Zhang HJ, Zhao W, Venkataraman S, et al. Activation of matrix metalloproteinase-2 by overexpression of manganese superoxide dismutase in human breast cancer MCF-7 cells involves reactive oxygen species. J Biol Chem 2002;277(23): 20919–26.

[70] Shariftabrizi A, Khorramizadeh MR, Saadat F, et al. Concomitant reduction of matrix metalloproteinase-2 secretion and intracellular reactive oxygen species following anti-sense inhibition of telomerase activity in PC-3 prostate carcinoma cells. Mol Cell Biochem 2005;273(1–2):109–16.

[71] Marsolais D, Cote CH, Frenette J. Nonsteroidal anti-inflammatory drug reduces neutrophil and macrophage accumulation but does not improve tendon regeneration. Lab Invest 2003;83(7):991–9.

[72] Simmons DL, Botting RM, Hla T. Cyclooxygenase isozymes: the biology of prostaglandin synthesis and inhibition. Pharmacol Rev 2004;56(3): 387–437.

[73] Hussain T, Gupta S, Mukhtar H. Cyclooxygenase-2 and prostate carcinogenesis. Cancer Lett 2003; 191(2):125–35.

[74] Tsatsanis C, Androulidaki A, Venihaki M, et al. Signalling networks regulating cyclooxygenase-2. Int J Biochem Cell Biol 2006;38(10):1654–61.

[75] Zha S, Yegnasubramanian V, Nelson WG, et al. Cyclooxygenases in cancer: progress and perspective. Cancer Lett 2004;215(1):1–20.

[76] Subbarayan V, Sabichi AL, Llansa N, et al. Differential expression of cyclooxygenase-2 and its regulation by tumor necrosis factor-alpha in normal and malignant prostate cells. Cancer Res 2001; 61(6):2720–6.

[77] Munoz-Espada AC, Watkins BA. Cyanidin attenuates PGE2 production and cyclooxygenase-2 expression in LNCaP human prostate cancer cells. J Nutr Biochem 2006;17(9):589–96.

[78] Syeda F, Grosjean J, Houliston RA, et al. Cyclooxygenase-2 induction and prostacyclin release by protease-activated receptors in endothelial cells

require cooperation between mitogen-activated protein kinase and NF-kappaB pathways. J Biol Chem 2006;281(17):11792–804.

[79] Lappas M, Yee K, Permezel M, et al. Lipopolysaccharide and TNF-alpha activate the nuclear factor kappa B pathway in the human placental JEG-3 cells. Placenta 2006;27(6–7):568–75.

[80] Choi JK, Lee SG, Lee JY, et al. Silica induces human cyclooxygenase-2 gene expression through the NF-kappaB signaling pathway. J Environ Pathol Toxicol Oncol 2005;24(3):163–74.

[81] Wang W, Bergh A, Damber JE. Chronic inflammation in benign prostate hyperplasia is associated with focal upregulation of cyclooxygenase-2, Bcl-2, and cell proliferation in the glandular epithelium. Prostate 2004;61(1):60–72.

[82] Matthias C, Schuster MT, Zieger S, et al. COX-2 inhibitors celecoxib and rofecoxib prevent oxidative DNA fragmentation. Anticancer Res 2006; 26(3A):2003–7.

[83] Wang W, Bergh A, Damber JE. Cyclooxygenase-2 expression correlates with local chronic inflammation and tumor neovascularization in human prostate cancer. Clin Cancer Res 2005;11(9):3250–6.

[84] Lee LM, Pan CC, Cheng CJ, et al. Expression of cyclooxygenase-2 in prostate adenocarcinoma and benign prostatic hyperplasia. Anticancer Res 2001;21(2B):1291–4.

[85] Yoshimura R, Sano H, Masuda C, et al. Expression of cyclooxygenase-2 in prostate carcinoma. Cancer 2000;89(3):589–96.

[86] Gupta S, Srivastava M, Ahmad N, et al. Overexpression of cyclooxygenase-2 in human prostate adenocarcinoma. Prostate 2000;42(1):73–8.

[87] Jin TX, Li XG, Wu WY, et al. [Expression of cyclooxygenase-2 and vascular endothelial growth factor in human prostate cancer and its significance]. Zhonghua Nan Ke Xue 2006;12(3):207–10 [in Chinese].

[88] Uotila P, Valve E, Martikainen P, et al. Increased expression of cyclooxygenase-2 and nitric oxide synthase-2 in human prostate cancer. Urol Res 2001;29(1):23–8.

[89] Zha S, Gage WR, Sauvageot J, et al. Cyclooxygenase-2 is up-regulated in proliferative inflammatory atrophy of the prostate, but not in prostate carcinoma. Cancer Res 2001;61(24):8617–23.

[90] Cohen BL, Gomez P, Omori Y, et al. Cyclooxygenase-2 (COX-2) expression is an independent predictor of prostate cancer recurrence. Int J Cancer 2006;119(5):1082–7.

[91] Liu XH, Kirschenbaum A, Yao S, et al. Inhibition of cyclooxygenase-2 suppresses angiogenesis and the growth of prostate cancer in vivo. J Urol 2000;164(3 Pt 1):820–5.

[92] Liu XH, Kirschenbaum A, Lu M, et al. Prostaglandin E(2) stimulates prostatic intraepithelial neoplasia cell growth through activation of the interleukin-6/GP130/STAT-3 signaling pathway.

Biochem Biophys Res Commun 2002;290(1): 249–55.

[93] Farivar-Mohseni H, Kandzari SJ, Zaslau S, et al. Synergistic effects of Cox-1 and -2 inhibition on bladder and prostate cancer in vitro. Am J Surg 2004;188(5):505–10.

[94] Fujita H, Koshida K, Keller ET, et al. Cyclooxygenase-2 promotes prostate cancer progression. Prostate 2002;53(3):232–40.

[95] Yuan A, Yu CJ, Shun CT, et al. Total cyclooxygenase-2 mRNA levels correlate with vascular endothelial growth factor mRNA levels, tumor angiogenesis and prognosis in non-small cell lung cancer patients. Int J Cancer 2005;115(4):545–55.

[96] Kirschenbaum A, Liu X, Yao S, et al. The role of cyclooxygenase-2 in prostate cancer. Urology 2001;58(2 Suppl 1):127–31.

[97] Pereg D, Lishner M. Non-steroidal anti-inflammatory drugs for the prevention and treatment of cancer. J Intern Med 2005;258(2):115–23.

[98] Liu CH, Chang SH, Narko K, et al. Overexpression of cyclooxygenase-2 is sufficient to induce tumorigenesis in transgenic mice. J Biol Chem 2001; 276(21):18563–9.

[99] Liu XH, Yao S, Kirschenbaum A, et al. NS398, a selective cyclooxygenase-2 inhibitor, induces apoptosis and down-regulates bcl-2 expression in LNCaP cells. Cancer Res 1998;58(19):4245–9.

[100] Dandekar DS, Lokeshwar BL. Inhibition of cyclooxygenase (COX)-2 expression by Tet-inducible COX-2 antisense cDNA in hormone-refractory prostate cancer significantly slows tumor growth and improves efficacy of chemotherapeutic drugs. Clin Cancer Res 2004;10(23):8037–47.

[101] Huh J, Liepins A, Zielonka J, et al. Cyclooxygenase 2 rescues LNCaP prostate cancer cells from sanguinarine-induced apoptosis by a mechanism involving inhibition of nitric oxide synthase activity. Cancer Res 2006;66(7):3726–36.

[102] Corcoran CA, He Q, Huang Y, et al. Cyclooxygenase-2 interacts with p53 and interferes with p53-dependent transcription and apoptosis. Oncogene 2005;24(9):1634–40.

[103] Attiga FA, Fernandez PM, Weeraratna AT, et al. Inhibitors of prostaglandin synthesis inhibit human prostate tumor cell invasiveness and reduce the release of matrix metalloproteinases. Cancer Res 2000;60(16):4629–37.

[104] Harris RE, Beebe-Donk J, Doss H, et al. Aspirin, ibuprofen, and other non-steroidal anti-inflammatory drugs in cancer prevention: a critical review of non-selective COX-2 blockade [review]. Oncol Rep 2005;13(4):559–83.

[105] Roberts RO, Jacobson DJ, Girman CJ, et al. A population-based study of daily nonsteroidal anti-inflammatory drug use and prostate cancer. Mayo Clin Proc 2002;77(3):219–25.

[106] Nelson JE, Harris RE. Inverse association of prostate cancer and non-steroidal anti-inflammatory

drugs (NSAIDs): results of a case-control study. Oncol Rep 2000;7(1):169–70.

[107] Mahmud S, Franco E, Aprikian A. Prostate cancer and use of nonsteroidal anti-inflammatory drugs: systematic review and meta-analysis. Br J Cancer 2004;90(1):93–9.

[108] Garcia Rodriguez LA, Gonzalez-Perez A. Inverse association between nonsteroidal anti-inflammatory drugs and prostate cancer. Cancer Epidemiol Biomarkers Prev 2004;13(4):649–53.

[109] Menezes RJ, Swede H, Niles R, et al. Regular use of aspirin and prostate cancer risk (United States). Cancer Causes Control 2006;17(3):251–6.

[110] Bosetti C, Talamini R, Negri E, et al. Aspirin and the risk of prostate cancer. Eur J Cancer Prev 2006;15(1):43–5.

[111] Liu X, Plummer SJ, Nock NL, et al. Nonsteroidal anti-inflammatory drugs and decreased risk of advanced prostate cancer: modification by lymphotoxin alpha. Am J Epidemiol 2006;164(10):984–9.

[112] Dasgupta K, Di CD, Ghosn J, et al. Association between nonsteroidal anti-inflammatory drugs and prostate cancer occurrence. Cancer J 2006;12(2): 130–5.

[113] Mahmud SM, Tanguay S, Begin LR, et al. Non-steroidal anti-inflammatory drug use and prostate cancer in a high-risk population. Eur J Cancer Prev 2006;15(2):158–64.

[114] Jacobs EJ, Rodriguez C, Mondul AM, et al. A large cohort study of aspirin and other nonsteroidal anti-inflammatory drugs and prostate cancer incidence. J Natl Cancer Inst 2005;97(13): 975–80.

[115] Pruthi RS, Derksen JE, Moore D. A pilot study of use of the cyclooxygenase-2 inhibitor celecoxib in recurrent prostate cancer after definitive radiation therapy or radical prostatectomy. BJU Int 2004; 93(3):275–8.

[116] Pruthi RS, Derksen JE, Moore D, et al. Phase II trial of celecoxib in prostate-specific antigen recurrent prostate cancer after definitive radiation therapy or radical prostatectomy. Clin Cancer Res 2006;12(7 Pt 1):2172–7.

[117] Smith MR, Manola J, Kaufman DS, et al. Celecoxib versus placebo for men with prostate cancer and a rising serum prostate-specific antigen after radical prostatectomy and/or radiation therapy. J Clin Oncol 2006;24(18):2723–8.

ELSEVIER
SAUNDERS

Urol Clin N Am 35 (2008) 131–136

UROLOGIC
CLINICS
of North America

Index

Note: Page numbers of article titles are in **boldface** type.

0094-0143/08/$ - see front matter © 2008 Elsevier Inc. All rights reserved.
doi:10.1016/S0094-0143(07)00125-5

urologic.theclinics.com

Moving?

Make sure your subscription moves with you!

To notify us of your new address, find your **Clinics Account Number** (located on your mailing label above your name), and contact customer service at:

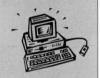

E-mail: elspcs@elsevier.com

800-654-2452 (subscribers in the U.S. & Canada)
407-345-4000 (subscribers outside of the U.S. & Canada)

Fax number: 407-363-9661

Elsevier Periodicals Customer Service
6277 Sea Harbor Drive
Orlando, FL 32887-4800

*To ensure uninterrupted delivery of your subscription, please notify us at least 4 weeks in advance of move.